THE LIVER DISORDERS SOURCEBOOK

THE LIVER DISORDERS SOURCEBOOK

Howard J. Worman, M.D.

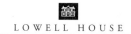

LOWELL HOUSE

LOS ANGELES

NTC/Contemporary Publishing Group

Library of Congress Cataloging-in-Publication Data

Worman, Howard J.
    The liver disorders sourcebook / by Howard J. Worman.
        p.   cm.
    Includes bibliographical references and index.
    ISBN 0-7373-0090-6
    1. Liver—Diseases Popular works.   I. Title.
RC845.W67   1999
616.3'62—dc21   99-24103
                                                     CIP

Published by Lowell House

A division of NTC/Contemporary Publishing Group, Inc.

4255 West Touhy Avenue, Lincolnwood (Chicago), Illinois 60646-1975 U.S.A.

Copyright©1999 by NTC/Contemporary Publishing Group, Inc.

Printed in the United States of America

International Standard Book Number: 0-7373-0090-6

01 02 03 04 RRD 18 17 16 15 14 13 12 11 10 9 8 7 6 5 4 3

To Terry

Contents

Preface

All of my previously published works have been in medical or scientific journals. In 1995, however, I started the Diseases of the Liver World Wide Website (http://cpmcnet.columbia.edu/dept/gi/disliv.html). This website has become a popular resource, accessed mostly by patients with liver diseases, their families, and their friends.

From reading numerous e-mail messages transmitted by users, I realized that thousands of individuals are seeking a responsible source of information on liver diseases, though few are available. Furthermore, it seems as if most doctors have a hard time explaining those liver diseases which often produce symptoms that, to the lay person, are not obviously related to the liver. So when Lowell House suggested I write a book on the subject, I accepted the offer to put together a text resource on liver diseases for patients, their families, and concerned friends.

The material in this book is primarily for the lay person. Some health professionals who are involved in the care of patients with liver disorders will hopefully find it very useful also. Its aim is to help the reader develop an understanding of what the liver does, what goes wrong during various diseases, what a doctor thinks when seeing patients with liver diseases, and what treatments are available. This book is certainly *not* a substitute for professional medical care. The reader *must* realize that specific diagnostic and treatment recommendations *can be made only by an experienced physician who knows the patient's complete history.*

This book is also not meant to be a comprehensive or exhaustive description of liver diseases. Some are remarkably complex and, out of necessity, I have simplified certain aspects for easy comprehension. However, because of the complexity of some liver diseases, I also felt it was incumbent to include brief discussions of virology, immunology, and genetics in some sections. I have tried my best to make these discussions as uncomplicated as possible. Readers who want to skip them will still glean some understanding of the various liver diseases. Readers who are fascinated by these basic aspects of disease will, hopefully, be stimulated to look elsewhere to learn more.

Being trained as an internist and not as a pediatrician, I apologize if there are details lacking from the discussions of liver diseases that uniquely affect infants and children. For interested readers who would like more details, I have included a bibliography of more complete resources and medical references. I have also included contact information for legitimate support groups and organizations that provide information for patients with liver diseases.

Several individuals have been helpful in the conception of this book from start to finish. My mother and father, Dora and Louis Worman, put me through college and medical school and provided me with the education that made this work possible. Dr. Fenton Schaffner, George Baher Professor Emeritus of Medicine at the Mount Sinai School of Medicine, taught me how to be a liver specialist, and without his expertise I probably could not have written this book. I thank Edwin Baum for providing important legal advice and Arlene M. Sklar and Louis Worman for help with business matters. My frequent discussions with Dr. Howard P. Reynolds while writing the book were also, as always, very interesting. Finally, Bud Sperry at Lowell House provided invaluable editing assistance, and Terry Chun supported me throughout this project.

Howard J. Worman
New York, NY

CHAPTER 1

The Normal Liver

Virtually everybody knows that the liver is an organ essential to life, but when most people are asked what the liver does, they do not know. Many will say that the liver plays some role in "purifying" or "cleansing" the blood. Some will know that it is the site of metabolism for many different drugs. Others will know that the liver is involved in the formation of bile.

The liver has many different functions, indeed. A thorough understanding of the three critical aspects of normal liver structure and function is essential to understanding what has gone wrong in a diseased liver. The first critical aspect is the liver's overall anatomy, in particular its blood supply. The second aspect is the synthetic biochemical functioning of the hepatocytes, the predominant cells in the liver. The third critical aspect is the central role of the liver in the metabolism and secretion of bilirubin.

Anatomy and Blood Supply

The liver is located in the right upper quadrant of the abdomen (Figure 1.1). If you place your fingers under your rib cage on the right side, you should be able to feel the edge of your liver when you take a deep breath. The liver itself is divided into the right and left lobes plus smaller lobes called the caudate and quadrate lobes. Various ligaments separate the lobes from each other. Most of the liver's mass is found in the right lobe. The entire surface of the liver is covered by a capsule that contains nerves that can sense pain. The gallbladder is located under the liver.

Familiarity with the blood supply of the liver is essential to understanding its function as well as some of the major complications of cirrhosis (chapter 3). About one-quarter of a person's blood volume passes through the liver every minute. How this blood supply is delivered to the liver is outlined in Figure 1.2.

The liver receives most of its blood from the portal vein. Blood from the portal vein does not reach the liver directly from the heart but passes first through the gut. Because of this, the liver is the first organ to gain nutrients, drugs, and toxins that are absorbed from the stomach and intestine. As a result, the liver plays a primary role in their metabolism. The portal vein also connects with the splenic vein, which drains the spleen. The connection between portal vein and splenic vein is important because if the blood flow to, within, or exiting the liver is impeded for any reason, it will back up into the spleen.

The liver also receives blood from the hepatic artery. Blood in the hepatic artery reaches the liver directly from the heart after passing through the lungs and is higher in oxygen content than the blood in the portal vein. The blood from the portal

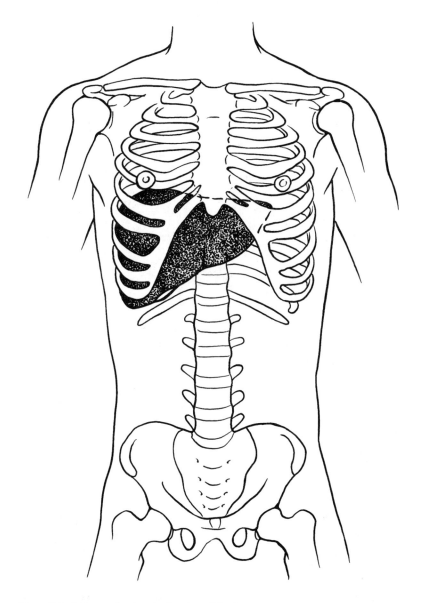

Figure 1.1. *Diagram showing the location of the liver.*
Illustration by Elizabeth Weadon Massari

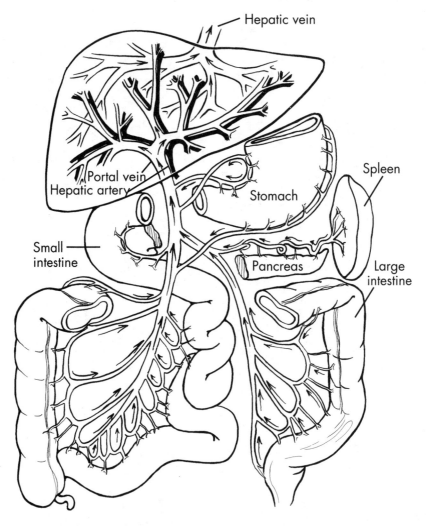

Hepatic vein

Portal vein
Hepatic artery

Stomach

Spleen

Small
intestine

Pancreas

Large
intestine

Figure 1.2. *Diagram showing the liver's blood supply.*

Blood enters the liver via the hepatic artery and portal vein. The
blood from the hepatic artery is oxygen-rich and comes directly from
the heart, whereas the blood in the portal vein has already absorbed
nutrients and other substances from the gastrointestinal tract. Within
the liver, the blood supplies from these two vessels mix. Blood leaves
the liver via the hepatic vein, which drains into the vena cava, which
returns the blood to the heart.

Illustration by Elizabeth Weadon Massari

vein and hepatic artery mix when entering the liver. The dual blood supply to the liver makes the probability of suffering an infarction (or death of tissue due to loss of blood supply from a clot such as occurs in the heart during a myocardial infarction, or heart attack) low.

Within the liver itself, blood flows through specialized capillaries called sinusoids. The sinusoids are quite permeable and allow compounds in the blood to have direct access to hepatocytes, which are the major cells of the liver. Many nutrients, drugs, and toxins in the blood are readily transported through the walls of the sinusoids and taken up by the hepatocytes where they are metabolized.

Blood exits the liver via the hepatic vein. From the hepatic vein, the blood enters the body's largest vein, the vena cava, and returns to the heart. A small amount of blood flow to the liver may never have access to the hepatocytes and returns directly to the heart via the hepatic vein.

Biochemical Functions of Liver Cells

The liver performs numerous biochemical functions. These functions take place primarily in the hepatocytes, which are the predominant cells in the liver. Some of the most important biochemical functions of the liver are:

- Synthesis of blood clotting factors
- Metabolism of alcohol and many drugs
- Detoxification of various harmful substances
- Conjugation and secretion of bilirubin

- Synthesis of bile salts
- Glucose (simple sugar) and carbohydrate (complex sugar) metabolism
- Cholesterol and fatty acid metabolism
- Protein metabolism

The liver synthesizes several factors involved in blood clotting, and normal function is necessary to prevent bleeding. Another function is synthesis and secretion of albumin, the major protein present in the blood. Albumin is necessary for maintaining proper fluid balance; decreases in blood albumin concentration can contribute to abnormal accumulation of fluid in the body. The synthesis of clotting factors and albumin are two of the most important biochemical functions of the liver and they are frequently assessed when diagnosing and treating patients with liver disorders.

The liver is the site of metabolism of many nutrients. Carbohydrates, fats, and proteins are all broken down and synthesized there. Normal liver function is critical for maintaining adequate blood sugar concentrations. The liver is also the major site of ammonia metabolism. Ammonia is a nitrogen compound that primarily results from the metabolism of proteins. If liver function is abnormal, poor mental functioning can result because ammonia, and probably other nitrogen compounds, is not adequately metabolized.

Because most compounds absorbed from the gastrointestinal tract pass through the liver first before reaching the systemic circulation, the liver is the organ of "first pass" metabolism of many drugs. Many compounds present in the environment, some of which are toxins, are also first metabolized in the liver. Metabolism in the liver usually leads to detoxification of environmental compounds, hence the concept that the liver "purifies" or "cleanses" the blood. The detoxified metabolites are then eliminated from the body, by either kidney secretion into the urine or secretion into the bile by the liver. Sometimes, liver metabolism can lead to the production of metabolites that are more toxic than the parent drug or environmental toxin itself. One example is carbon tetrachloride, which is metabolized in the liver and becomes an extremely toxic compound that kills liver cells.

Bilirubin Formation and Secretion

Bilirubin derives primarily from the breakdown of old red blood cells (a small fraction also comes from the breakdown of proteins in other organs). Dying red blood cells (the life span of a normal red blood cell is approximately 120 days) are taken up by specialized cells—primarily in the spleen—where they are destroyed. The major red blood cell protein hemoglobin, which is the protein that carries oxygen in the blood, is then chemically converted to bilirubin, which is greenish yellow in color.

Bilirubin is extremely insoluble in water and circulates in the bloodstream bound to albumin. Albumin-bound bilirubin is taken up from the blood by hepatocytes. In hepatocytes, bilirubin is chemically converted by a process called *conjugation* into an increased water-soluble form. In conjugation, bilirubin undergoes a chemical reaction with a water-soluble compound called glucuronic acid. As a result of this chemical reaction, two glucuronic acid molecules are usually attached to one bilirubin molecule. The result is a compound known as bilirubin diglucuronide. Bilirubin diglucuronide is generally referred to as conjugated bilirubin. (Actually, a rather small amount of conjugated bilirubin has only one glucuronic acid molecule attached and is known as bilirubin monoglucuronide.) The bilirubin conjugation reaction normally proceeds extremely slowly, but in the liver it is catalyzed (sped up) due to an enzyme known as UDP–glucuronosyltransferase. Without this enzyme, bilirubin conjugation does not occur to any appreciable degree.

Conjugated bilirubin is secreted from the hepatocytes into the very tiny bile ducts within the liver. These tiny ducts merge into larger bile ducts that eventually form the common bile duct that empties into the small intestine. In the healthy liver, almost all of the conjugated bilirubin is secreted into the common bile duct and only a very small amount leaks out of hepatocytes and back into the bloodstream. As a result of conjugation in the liver and secretion into the bile, the total blood bilirubin concentration in normal individuals is usually less than 1 mg per deciliter. The steps in bilirubin metabolism and secretion are outlined in Figure 1.3.

When bilirubin in the blood is measured in the clinical laboratory, values for *direct* and *total* bilirubin are usually reported. The direct bilirubin represents roughly the more water-soluble conjugated bilirubin. The direct bilirubin measured in the clinical laboratory is normally only one-third or less of total bilirubin in the blood. Actually, there is much less conjugated bilirubin in the blood than the amount of direct bilirubin measured in the clinical laboratory. Because of the methodology routinely applied, the concentration of conjugated or direct bilirubin in the blood is usually overestimated. This is not significant as this overestimation is always accounted for in the normal values. Most of the total bilirubin in the blood is the unconjugated bilirubin produced from hemoglobin and other proteins prior to being conjugated in the liver. The estimate of the unconjugated bilirubin measured either in the clinical laboratory, or calculated as total bilirubin minus direct bilirubin, is called *indirect* bilirubin.

The conversion of compounds to more water-soluble forms by conjugation in the liver is a general process that also plays a

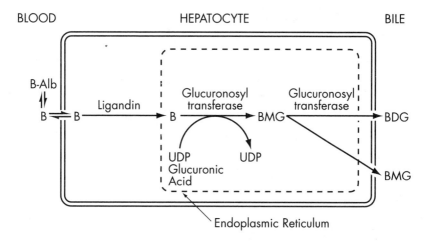

Figure 1.3. *Schematic diagram outlining the metabolism of bilirubin to the liver.*
Albumin-bound bilirubin is taken by hepatocytes from the blood.
In hepatocytes, bilirubin may be transiently bound to a compound
called ligandin. The bilirubin is conjugated to glucuronic acid
within the endoplasmic reticulum of the hepatocyte. The enzyme
UDP–glucuronosyltransferase helps this chemical reaction take place.
The conjugated bilirubin (primarily bilirubin diglucuronide [BDG]
and a small amount of bilirubin monoglucoronide [BMG]) is secreted
from the hepatocytes into the bile.

role in metabolism of compounds other than bilirubin. Drugs
and toxins are frequently conjugated to glucuronic acid and become more water soluble, thus facilitating elimination from the
body. Several slightly different forms of the enzyme UDP–glucuronosyltransferase are responsible for conjugation of different
compounds with glucuronic acid. In addition, some drugs and
toxins are conjugated to other water-soluble chemical moieties,
such as sulfate, for secretion from the body.

Conjugated bilirubin, or other conjugated compounds, that leak out from the liver into the blood are, generally, filtered readily by the kidneys and secreted in the urine. If the concentration of conjugated bilirubin in the blood becomes too high, it can be detected in the urine. If the liver for some reason fails to secrete conjugated bilirubin into the bile, the urine may appear dark yellow or brown.

Critical Things to Remember About Liver Structure and Function

Before reading any further, it is essential to keep in mind the following aspects of normal liver structure and function:

- The liver receives most of its blood from the portal vein. This blood passes first through the gut and is rich in materials absorbed from the stomach and intestine. The portal vein is also connected to the splenic vein.
- The liver is the first site of metabolism of many nutrients, drugs, and toxins.
- Hepatocytes, the predominant cells in the liver, perform many biochemical functions that are essential for normal life. Two critical biochemical functions of the liver assessed in diagnosing and following patients with liver diseases are the synthesis of blood clotting factors and the synthesis of albumin.
- The liver takes unconjugated bilirubin from the blood and conjugates it to a more water-soluble form that is secreted into the bile. The amount of bilirubin in the blood normally does not exceed 1 mg per deciliter.

CHAPTER 2

The Diseased Liver

When the Liver Is Affected by Disease

Liver disease affects the normal functions of the liver. Abnormalities in liver function, however, are usually *not* apparent in most individuals with chronic liver disease until the disease is rather advanced. Clinical and laboratory evidence of abnormal function is usually not present unless the liver is significantly compromised. Patients with clinically abnormal liver function usually have advanced cirrhosis or acute destruction of liver cells (discussed in chapter 3). Nevertheless, there are clinical findings and laboratory tests that can detect liver disease prior to significant deterioration in liver function. Before discussing these clinical finding and laboratory tests, however, it is important to distinguish *chronic* versus *acute* liver disease.

Acute Versus Chronic Disease

A critical distinction is to establish whether a liver disease is acute or chronic. Acute diseases occur suddenly and are usually relatively short in duration. Chronic diseases are typically long-term and their onset may be insidious. A general definition of a chronic liver disease is one lasting more than six months.

The concerns in acute and chronic liver disease are different to some extent. An acute liver disease either resolves itself, becomes chronic, or kills the patient. Some acute liver diseases can cause a severe type of liver failure known as *fulminant hepatic failure* (see chapter 3). The therapeutic goal in acute liver disease is to keep the patient alive and, if possible, to prevent the disease from becoming chronic. This involves either curing the acute disease or supporting the patient until it spontaneously resolves. The therapeutic goal in chronic liver disease is to either cure the disorder, prevent it from advancing, or control the complications. Preventing advancement of a chronic liver disease usually means stopping it from becoming cirrhosis. In an individual who already has cirrhosis, preventing further deterioration of liver function and controlling the resulting complications are the treatment goals.

Causes of Acute and Chronic Liver Disease

Several agents cause only acute liver disease:

- Hepatitis A virus
- Hepatitis E virus
- Other viral infections
- Overdose of some drugs
- Short-term exposure to some drugs and toxins
- Shock

Important examples are the hepatitis A virus and hepatitis E virus. Infection from these viruses never becomes chronic. Other viruses, such as yellow fever or dengue, can cause acute liver disease. Single or brief exposures to certain toxic substances, or single overdoses of some drugs such as acetaminophen, can also cause acute liver disease.

Some liver diseases are chronic by definition. There are chronic, congenital disorders, resulting from the inheritance of abnormal genes such as hemochromatosis, Wilson disease, and alpha-1-antitrypsin deficiency. Primary biliary cirrhosis and sclerosing cholangitis are also chronic diseases. Autoimmune hepatitis is always a chronic disease. Cirrhosis, which is identified by scarring and nodules in the liver, is a chronic disease and occurs after long-term damage to the liver from inflammation or other insults.

Several agents can cause both acute and chronic hepatitis:

- Alcohol
- Many drugs
- Hepatitis B virus
- Hepatitis C virus
- Hepatitis D virus (only in individuals with hepatitis B)
- Circulatory problems (e.g., heart failure)

Drinking alcohol heavily for several weeks, for example, can cause acute fatty liver or hepatitis that will resolve if the individual stops drinking. However, most alcohol-induced liver disease is chronic as most alcohol abusers drink for years. There are several other drugs and toxins in addition to alcohol that can cause both acute and chronic liver disease.

The hepatitis B virus can cause both acute and chronic hepatitis. About 90 percent of adults infected with hepatitis B virus develop acute liver disease that resolves or, in about 2 percent of cases, kills the patient if liver transplantation is not performed. About 5 percent of adults acutely infected with hepatitis B virus develop chronic hepatitis (hepatitis that lasts longer than six months). In newborn babies, the situation is virtually opposite that of adults, as about 90 percent of infants acutely infected with hepatitis B virus at or near birth become infected for life. About 85 percent of individuals infected with hepatitis C virus develop chronic hepatitis. In rare cases, the hepatitis C virus can cause acute liver disease. In most cases, however, the acute infection is asymptomatic.

Problems in Establishing Acute from Chronic Liver Disease

Although obvious on the surface, the distinction between acute and chronic liver disease is not always straightforward. A patient with a chronic liver disease that has not been diagnosed at an earlier stage may present to the doctor with worsening, or newly apparent, symptoms or laboratory abnormalities. Examples could be Wilson disease, autoimmune hepatitis, or hemochromatosis. In other instances, patients with cirrhosis can have acute worsening of liver function if, for example, they become infected. Such a case can be considered an acute exacerbation, or acute presentation, of a chronic disease.

Patients with acute liver diseases can often be misdiagnosed as having chronic liver diseases. Patients with severe, acute alcoholic or viral hepatitis, for example, sometimes have the same signs and symptoms as patients with end-stage cirrhosis and can be misdiagnosed as having cirrhosis. In these cases, the illness and symptoms can resolve completely. An acute liver disease can also occur superimposed on a chronic liver disease. For example, individuals with cirrhosis—a chronic disease—can develop acute hepatitis on top of the existing cirrhosis. A classic example is the alcoholic with cirrhosis whose condition suddenly worsens when developing acute alcoholic hepatitis from binge drinking. The doctor must keep all of these possibilities in mind when approaching a patient with a liver disease, especially one seeking medical attention for the first time.

A Patient with Liver Disease Visits the Doctor

The diagnosis of liver diseases depends upon a combination of history, physical examination, laboratory tests, radiological tests (usually), and frequently a liver biopsy. It is hazardous to accurately diagnose a liver disease without knowing all of this information. Individuals often call or send me e-mail messages with one or two test results and ask, "What's wrong?" My standard answer is, "Only a doctor who obtains a complete history, examines the patient, reviews all of the laboratory test results, knows the results of relevant radiological tests, and, in some cases, examines the liver biopsy can make an accurate diagnosis of liver disease." Having emphasized this fact, I will review the aspects of history, physical examination, laboratory tests, radiological tests, and liver biopsy relevant to the diagnosis of individuals with liver diseases. The following information should provide patients with a general idea about what to expect when they see their doctors.

History

As in any medical specialty or subspecialty, a cornerstone of the diagnosis of liver disease is the patient's history. There are certain historical facts that are of primary importance in diagnosing a patient with suspected liver disease. Patients should be willing to openly discuss the following issues with their doctors:

- Honest assessment of alcohol consumption
- Careful assessment of prescription and over-the-counter drug use
- Intravenous drug use, *even if only once long ago*
- Sexual activities
- Blood transfusions
- Travel to or emigration from certain areas of the world
- Exposure to possible environmental toxins
- Ingestion of contaminated foods
- Liver disease in family members

Drug and alcohol use must be carefully evaluated in a patient with liver disease. Alcohol abuse is the leading cause of acquired liver disease in the United States and most Western countries. Patients should not hide information from or lie to their doctors about the amount of alcohol they drink (nonetheless, virtually all individuals with alcohol abuse or dependence disorders significantly underreport alcohol consumption). The quantity of alcohol that individuals must consume to acquire liver disease varies tremendously; the reasons for these differences are unknown. Some individuals can drink half a gallon of alcohol a day and never develop liver disease (they will likely develop several other medical problems!) while others may develop liver disease from drinking as little as two drinks per day over many years. In general, alcohol should always be considered as a possible contributing factor to liver disease in individuals who regularly consume more than two drinks per day.

Both prescription and over-the-counter drugs can cause liver disease. It is essential for an examining doctor to obtain a thorough drug history from individuals with suspected liver disease and for patients to discuss all drug use in detail with their doctors. Even if drugs are not the cause of liver disease, drugs may be metabolized differently in patients with liver disease and can contribute to an underlying problem. Toxins and even unusual food products, such as Jamaican bush tea or *Amanita phalloides* mushrooms, can also cause liver disease.

Viruses that cause acute and chronic hepatitis are spread by various routes, and information about possible exposure is of vital importance to any medical history. Hepatitis B, C, and D viruses are spread by blood and blood products, and important information includes knowledge of past blood transfusions and past or present intravenous drug use. Even someone who used intravenous drugs *just once* in the remote past could be infected with the hepatitis B or C virus; thus, patients should openly discuss any prior drug use with their doctors. Questions about sex can be embarrassing, but a careful history of sexual practices is also important as hepatitis viruses, especially hepatitis B virus, can be transmitted by homosexual and heterosexual relations.

Hepatitis A is generally transmitted by contaminated foods—usually seafood—or unsanitary conditions of waste disposal. If a patient presents with acute liver disease, it is important to rule out this virus as a cause and obtain a careful history of food consumption. A travel history is also important to detect travel to countries where hepatitis A is common, or to parts of the world where infection due to hepatitis E virus occurs. A history of living in certain countries in Asia, or parts of Africa where hepatitis B infection is endemic, should also be ascertained. Past or present occupational exposure to blood products, for example, employment or volunteer work in the health care field, should also be investigated.

Several liver diseases are inherited. For this reason, it is important to ask a patient with suspected liver disease about family history. A family history may also be relevant to liver diseases that are not inherited. For example, a careful family history may identify a household contact with viral hepatitis that could prove contagious.

Many individuals with liver disease will have no symptoms or only nonspecific complaints such as fatigue or depression; other symptoms, however, are very suggestive of liver disease. A history of current or past jaundice (yellow skin and eyes) would be suggestive of liver disease. Itching, generally all over the body, could also be suggestive of liver dysfunction. Swelling in the abdomen and/or legs caused by fluid retention could be from cirrhosis. Confusion, from mild to severe, can also occur due to cirrhosis or acute liver failure. Bruising easily and bleeding upon even slight contact with objects may also indicate abnormal liver function. A doctor should question any patient with suspected liver disease about such symptoms.

Physical Examination

All patients with suspected liver disease should undergo a complete physical. Many, or even perhaps most, patients with liver disease will have a normal physical examination. There are several physical signs that can indicate the presence of liver disease or the severity of liver dysfunction. The physical examination begins with "inspection." Signs of liver disease may be apparent to the examining doctor just by looking at a patient. Jaundice may be obvious. Evidence of muscle wasting or weight loss may be obvious in the patient with cirrhosis. Severe fluid retention in the abdomen may also be readily visible in patients with advanced cirrhosis or severe, more recent liver damage.

Every patient with liver disease should be weighed. Obese individuals are at increased risk for fatty liver. Fluid retention in cirrhosis can lead to weight gain and weight should be regularly followed in individuals with cirrhosis. Weight loss may also occur in individuals who suffer from chronic liver abnormalities.

The doctor should also pay careful attention to specific parts of the physical examination that may indicate the presence of liver disease. The patient's hands should be examined for Depuytren's contracture, a shortening and thickening under the skin of the palm that can cause the middle fingers to be bent. Some individuals with cirrhosis or alcohol liver disease may have this. Patients with liver disease may also have what is known as "liver palms," which are palms that are abnormally red in color.

Examination of the skin is critical in the evaluation of a patient with suspected liver disease. Jaundice, a yellowing of the skin and whites of the eyes, is caused by a high concentration of bilirubin in the blood and is a hallmark of liver disease. It can also occur, however, in non-liver diseases, such as those caused by increased red blood cell destruction. At high blood bilirubin concentrations, the skin may appear obviously yellow. Jaundice is sometimes more readily observed under the nails or in the gums than in the skin, especially in individuals with dark skin. The skin should also be examined for bruises. Some individuals with chronic or severe liver disease will also have small vascular skin lesions called "spiders," or more correctly, *spider angiomata*. These are usually found on the arms, shoulders, chest, and back (they are virtually never found below the waistline). Spider angiomata are small red dots with "legs" that radiate from the center (hence the name). They blanch when compressed and turn red again when pressure is released.

Examination of head and eyes should also be performed. Jaundice may first be apparent in the whites of the eyes before yellowing of the skin is detectable. The doctor should examine the eyes carefully. Some individuals with liver disease, especially those with alcoholic cirrhosis, may have enlarged parotid glands (the salivary glands on the side of the face).

Examination of the abdomen is of central importance in the patient with liver disease. Protrusion of the abdomen may result from fluid retention. Some individuals with cirrhosis will have an umbilical hernia that sticks out of the belly button and can be temporarily pushed in by the doctor. The doctor should feel for the edge of the liver on the upper right side of the abdomen under the ribs, as the liver may be enlarged or abnormal in texture. Similarly, the doctor should feel for the spleen on the left upper portion of the abdomen. The spleen should not be felt in normal individuals but may be swollen in patients with liver disease. The doctor should also "percuss" the liver, that is, drum on your abdomen. Percussion allows the size of the liver to be estimated.

The liver may be enlarged (hepatomegaly) in some diseases and shrunken in others. The doctor should feel around the abdomen for the presence of retained fluid, which can also be detected by percussion of the flanks, and look at the legs and ankles for evidence of fluid retention.

An examination of the nervous system is important in the patient with liver disease. Patients with severe acute liver disease or cirrhosis may have *hepatic encephalopathy,* which can cause mental changes. Mental changes due to hepatic encephalopathy can range from very subtle changes in mental status to deep coma. The first mental status change that usually occurs is the inability to construct simple objects, such as a six-point star. Patients with early hepatic encephalopathy may also have difficulty with "connect the dots" drawings similar to those that children do. In cases of severe hepatic encephalopathy, marked confusion can occur and patients may have a "liver flap" (asterexis) in which the hand drops when held up by the patient like the hand of a policeman stopping traffic.

Having reviewed the above physical signs, it must again be emphasized that most individuals with liver disease will have a normal physical examination. Nevertheless, a careful physical examination is mandatory, and a doctor really cannot know what's going on without performing one.

Blood Testing

Blood tests play an important role in the diagnosis of liver disease and in following patients with various liver disorders. Blood tests comprise only a part of the picture, however, and must be considered along with the patient's history and physical examination. Isolated laboratory test results usually have very little meaning outside of the entire clinical picture. Despite this fact, patients with liver disease (and sometimes doctors) too often focus a tremendous amount of concern—usually too much—on the meaning of isolated, abnormal laboratory test results. Most patients, and even some doctors, have a difficult time understanding the significance of laboratory tests in liver disease. Very frequently, too much weight is given to the absolute values and random fluctuations of laboratory test results. After cautioning again that *a particular laboratory test result means little outside of the complete history,* I will explain the relevance of various blood tests commonly used to assess patients with liver disease. Some of the relevant tests that usually comprise part of "routine" blood biochemistry panels are summarized in Table 2.1.

Table 2.1. *Routine blood tests relevant to individuals with liver diseases.*

Test	What's Measured	Significance
ALT (SGPT)	Enzyme activity	Elevated in many liver diseases. Rough estimate for hepatocyte death from inflammation or other causes.
AST (SGOT)	Enzyme activity	Same as ALT but also may be elevated in heart or muscle cell death. Usually two or more times higher than ALT in alcoholic hepatitis.
Alkaline phosphatase	Enzyme activity	Elevation suggests abnormality of large bile ducts outside of liver or tiny ones within. May be elevated in non-liver diseases, especially disorders of tumors or bone.
GGTP	Enzyme activity	Same as alkaline phosphatase but specific for bile ducts. May be elevated in normal individuals or alcohol drinkers without structural liver disease.
Bilirubin	Concentration	Elevated in many liver diseases, mostly bile duct obstruction, severe acute liver damage, or advanced cirrhosis. May be elevated in non-liver diseases such as those of red blood cells.
Albumin	Concentration	Decreased in severe liver disease. Usually decreased in end-stage cirrhosis. Can also be decreased in some kidney diseases, intestinal disorders, malnourishment, or any serious chronic disease.
Prothrombin time	Time	Increased in advanced cirrhosis or severe acute liver damage. May be elevated in blood clotting disorders not related to the liver.

Aminotransferases (ALT and AST)

Aminotransferases are enzymes that facilitate certain chemical reactions within cells. Two major aminotransferases are present in hepatocytes, the primary liver cells. These are alanine aminotransferase (ALT) and aspartate aminotransferase (AST). (The older names for these enzymes, still used by some doctors and clinical laboratories, were SGPT and SGOT, respectively.) ALT is present almost exclusively in hepatocytes while AST is present in cells of some other tissues, such as heart and skeletal muscle. ALT and AST leak out from dead or damaged cells and into the bloodstream. As a result, their activities (activity is a unit of measurement used by biochemists that is roughly proportional to amount) in the blood can be measured. In healthy individuals, the activities (amounts) of ALT and AST in the blood fall into normal ranges that vary slightly from one laboratory to another. When hepatocyte death is increased, as in hepatitis, ALT and AST leak out of dying cells at greater rates and their activities in the blood are increased. Elevations in blood ALT and AST activities *therefore suggest increased hepatocyte death.*

ALT and AST activities are measured on routine blood testing panels as indicators of possible liver disease. Some doctors and nurses refer to them as "liver enzymes." ALT and AST have also come to be known as "liver function tests." This is unfortunate because blood ALT and AST activities do not relate to the liver's *function.* The activities of these enzymes in the blood correlate roughly to the degree of ongoing liver cell death or damage, but not liver function.

In most cases of hepatocyte death, blood ALT and AST activities are both elevated to approximately equal levels. One notable exception is alcoholic hepatitis, where for reasons that are unclear, the blood AST activity is frequently more highly elevated than the ALT activity. Blood AST activity, but not ALT activity, can also be elevated in non-liver diseases such as heart attack and skeletal muscle damage as this enzyme is present in heart and muscle cells as well as in hepatocytes. Sometimes, only the blood ALT activity will be elevated in liver disease while AST activity remains normal.

Blood aminotransferase activities are elevated in many different liver diseases. In chronic hepatitis from any cause (e.g., viruses, drugs, alcohol), they are usually less than ten times normal. ALT and AST are also elevated in cases of acute liver cell necrosis (death) caused by shock, drugs, toxins, viral hepatitis, or other insults. In cases of massive liver cell death, in shock, for example, or after an overdose of a drug toxic to the liver, blood aminotransferase activities can be several hundred times normal immediately after the injury and then rapidly return to near normal in a few days.

The degree of elevation of blood AST and ALT activities roughly approximates the amount of liver cell death from inflammation or other causes. Some individuals with hepatitis can have significant inflammation on biopsy and only mild elevations of blood aminotransferase activities, however. In rare cases, some individuals will exhibit very high blood aminotransferase activities and only mild inflammation on liver biopsy. This is one reason why liver biopsy is usually essential to the evaluation of patients with chronic hepatitis.

The most important things to remember about blood AST and ALT activities are:

1. Blood AST and ALT activities are elevated in many different liver diseases where liver cell death from inflammation or other causes occurs. Elevations in blood ALT and AST activities are not specific for any particular diagnosis and further evaluation is necessary.
2. AST and ALT activities are not "liver function tests" despite common jargon used by doctors and patients. ALT and AST

activities can be very high in someone with acute liver cell death and reasonably good liver function who will completely recover. On the other hand, they can be normal in someone with end-stage cirrhosis and virtually no remaining liver function.

3. Elevations of blood aminotransferase activities strongly suggest the presence of liver disease and should be evaluated by a doctor.

4. In individuals with known chronic liver disease such as viral hepatitis, blood ALT and AST should be periodically followed as approximate markers of the amount of liver inflammation or liver cell death.

5. ALT and AST activities should be tested in people at risk for liver disease. Examples include those taking certain drugs that can affect the liver and people with a past history of injection drug use.

Alkaline Phosphatase and Gamma-glutamyltranspeptidase (GGTP)

Two other enzyme activities measured routinely in the blood are important to diagnosing liver disease. These are the alkaline phosphatase and GGTP activities. Alkaline phosphatase is found in many different cells including those lining the large bile ducts and very tiny bile ducts in the liver. Alkaline phosphatase is also present in cells of the kidney, intestine, bone, and placenta. Blood alkaline phosphatase activity can be elevated in disorders involving any of these tissues. GGTP, on the other hand, is present almost exclusively in the parts of the hepatocytes that secrete bile plus the bile duct cells.

Elevations in blood alkaline phosphatase and GGTP activities, especially in the setting of normal or only modestly elevated ALT and AST activities, suggest bile duct disease or abnormal bile flow. These can be diseases of either the large bile ducts outside the liver, for example, obstruction by a gallstone or cancer, or of the tiny bile ducts within the liver. Many drugs also cause stagnation of bile flow, or *cholestasis,* and resultant elevations in blood alkaline phosphatase and GGTP activities. In liver diseases not directly affecting the bile ducts, such as hepatitis or cirrhosis, blood alkaline phosphatase and GGTP activities may also be elevated. In these diseases, however, elevations are usually more modest and ALT and AST activities become elevated to a more significant degree when hepatocyte death predominates.

In contrast, liver diseases that primarily affect the bile ducts are characterized by more marked elevations in blood alkaline phosphatase and GGTP activities and only modestly elevated or normal blood ALT and AST activities.

Abnormally high blood alkaline phosphatase may also be seen in a patient with bone disease. In addition, blood alkaline phosphatase activity may be elevated in pregnancy as it is produced by the placenta. In these instances, blood GGTP activity should be normal. If blood alkaline phosphatase activity is elevated together with serum GGTP activity, bile duct or liver disease is the likely cause.

Elevations in only blood GGTP activity can be problematic to evaluate. GGTP activity is an extremely sensitive and variable test and may be elevated to some degree in virtually any liver disease. It can also be elevated in some normal individuals and people with very subtle and clinically insignificant liver abnormalities. GGTP is also induced by many drugs, including alcohol, and its activity in the blood may be increased in heavy drinkers. Isolated elevations in blood GGTP activity suggest early bile duct disorders, liver diseases, heavy alcohol use, or drug use. However, GGTP can also be elevated in the absence of meaningful liver disease. Only an experienced physician who knows a patient's entire history can determine if and how an isolated elevation in blood GGTP activity needs to be evaluated further.

As is the case with aminotransferase activities, elevations in blood alkaline phosphatase or GGTP activities are *not* diagnostic for any specific disease. Their elevations suggest disorders of the bile ducts or bile flow. They may also be elevated to a lesser degree than ALT and AST in liver diseases that primarily affect hepatocytes.

Bilirubin

An elevated concentration of bilirubin in the blood is known as *hyperbilirubinemia*. Hyperbilirubinemia occurs as a result of four problems: 1) increased production; 2) decreased uptake by the liver; 3) decreased conjugation; or 4) decreased secretion from the liver. The normal bilirubin concentration in the blood is approximately less than 1 mg per deciliter. When the blood bilirubin exceeds about 2 mg per deciliter, jaundice becomes apparent.

In disorders causing increased production of bilirubin, the *indirect* bilirubin concentration in the blood will be elevated. Increased bilirubin production results from conditions that cause increased destruction of red blood cells and not from liver diseases. In such conditions, the direct bilirubin concentration in the blood will be normal as long as liver function is not compromised.

Indirect bilirubin concentration in the blood is also primarily increased in conditions that cause decreased bilirubin uptake by the liver or decreased conjugation within the liver. Decreased bilirubin uptake by hepatocytes can be caused by some drugs, fasting, and infections. Serious problems with bilirubin conjugation almost always present in childhood. These conditions include hereditary diseases in which the enzyme that conjugates bilirubin is lacking or abnormal, and jaundice of premature babies in which conjugation of bilirubin is impaired.

Most acquired liver diseases in adults cause impairment in bilirubin secretion from liver cells that results in elevations primarily in the *direct* bilirubin concentration in the blood. In most chronic acquired liver diseases, the blood bilirubin concentration is usually normal until a significant amount of liver damage has occurred and cirrhosis is present. The rise in blood bilirubin concentration is roughly proportional to the amount of liver dysfunction. In acute liver diseases, the serum bilirubin concentration usually rises in proportion to the severity of liver damage.

Disorders that cause obstruction of the small and large bile ducts also cause elevations in the direct bilirubin concentration in the blood. Some drugs also impede bile flow in the liver and cause elevations in direct bilirubin concentration. In these disorders, the blood alkaline phosphatase and GGTP activities are usually elevated concurrently.

When the concentration of direct bilirubin in the blood becomes high, some of it is filtered by the kidneys. This excreted bilirubin turns the urine yellow or brown in color. Bilirubin can also be detected by urinalysis.

Albumin

Albumin is the most abundant protein in the bloodstream. It is synthesized in the liver and secreted into the blood. If liver function is abnormal, the blood albumin concentration may fall. This usually occurs in patients with cirrhosis who have moderate or advanced liver dysfunction. The albumin concentration in the blood can also be low in conditions other than liver diseases including serious malnutrition, kidney diseases, and rare forms of intestinal dysfunction. Low albumin concentration in the blood is sometimes referred to as *hypoalbuminemia*.

Prothrombin Time (PT)

When liver function is compromised, the synthesis of several blood clotting factors may be decreased. The prothrombin time, often called the "PT," is a blood clotting test that measures the function of several blood clotting factors. The prothrombin time is prolonged when blood concentrations of some of the clotting factors made by the liver are low. In chronic liver diseases, the prothrombin time is usually not significantly prolonged until cirrhosis has developed and the amount of liver damage is significant. In acute liver diseases, the prothrombin time can be prolonged due to severe liver damage and then return to normal as the patient recovers. The prothrombin time can also be prolonged in other conditions besides liver diseases, such as vitamin K deficiency (which can arise from malabsorption in some bile duct diseases) and inherited or acquired blood clotting disorders. Drugs, for example warfarin (Coumadin®), which is used therapeutically as an anticoagulant, can also prolong prothrombin time.

Complete Blood Count (CBC) and Platelet Count

The complete blood count (CBC) is an important laboratory test in patients with liver diseases. Although not specific for liver problems, abnormalities may be seen on the complete blood count in patients with liver diseases. Individuals with chronic liver disease, especially cirrhosis, can be anemic and have low serum hemoglobin concentrations and hematocrits, which are roughly proportional to the number of red blood cells. Patients with cirrhosis can also have decreased white blood cells counts (white blood cells are the cells that fight infection). On the other hand, the white blood cell count can be increased in individuals with acute inflammatory liver diseases such as viral or alcoholic hepatitis.

An important part of the complete blood count in individuals with liver disease is the platelet count. Platelets are the smallest of the blood cells and are involved in blood clotting. In individuals with cirrhosis or very severe, acute liver disease, the spleen can become enlarged as blood flow through the liver is impeded. Platelets may become trapped in the enlarged spleen and, as a result, the platelet count can fall. A low platelet count (thrombocytopenia) in a patient with chronic liver disease suggests the presence of cirrhosis. Low platelet counts are not specific for liver diseases, however, and can be observed in many different conditions.

Serum Protein Electrophoresis

Serum protein electrophoresis is an informative blood test for patients with liver disease. It is not routinely done by most physicians, however. In this test, the blood's major proteins are separated in an electric field and their concentrations measured. The serum proteins measured in this test are albumin, alpha-globulins, beta-globulins, and gamma-globulins. The result can provide clues to several diagnostic possibilities and also about the liver's function.

Ammonia

Blood ammonia concentrations can increase when the liver fails. Ammonia is absorbed from the intestine where it is generated by the breakdown of proteins by bacteria that live in the colon. Ammonia is not effectively removed from the blood by the failing liver or the liver with advanced cirrhosis. As a result, the concentration of ammonia in the blood increases.

Elevations in blood ammonia concentration very roughly correlate to the degree of hepatic encephalopathy. However, hepatic encephalopathy should be followed by physical signs and symptoms and not by serial determinations of the blood ammonia. Onetime determination of blood ammonia concentration will suggest that the liver may not be properly functioning if it is elevated. Blood ammonia concentrations can be elevated in conditions other than liver failure, including rare metabolic disorders.

Laboratory Tests of Specific Liver Diseases

Several blood tests are performed for the diagnosis of specific liver diseases. Specific tests for viral components in serum and antibodies against viruses are used to diagnose viral hepatitis. Tests for certain "autoantibodies" are useful in the diagnosis of autoimmune liver diseases. Measurements of various metabolic products or minerals are helpful in the diagnosis of inherited liver diseases. Some of the various laboratory tests for specific viral, autoimmune, and congenital liver diseases are outlined in Table 2.2. These tests are discussed in greater detail in subsequent chapters on the specific liver diseases.

Table 2.2. Some laboratory tests for specific viral, autoimmune, and congenital liver diseases. *

Condition	Test
Viral hepatitis	
Hepatitis A	Antibodies against viral proteins for past or current infection
Hepatitis B	Antibodies against viral proteins for evidence of past or current infection; test for viral protein or DNA in blood for current infection
Hepatitis C	Antibodies against viral proteins and presence of viral RNA in blood for current infection
Hepatitis D	Antibodies against viral proteins for current infection
Hepatitis E	Antibodies against viral proteins for past or current infection
Autoimmune diseases	
Autoimmune hepatitis	"Autoantibodies" against proteins from cell nuclei (antinuclear antibodies) and smooth muscle cells (antismooth muscle antibodies)
Primary biliary cirrhosis	"Autoantibodies" against proteins from mitochondria (antimitochondrial antibodies) and certain antinuclear antibodies
Primary sclerosing cholangitis	"Autoantibodies" known as "ANCA"
Congenital diseases	
Hemochromatosis	Iron, transferrin, and ferritin
Wilson disease	Ceruloplasmin, urine copper
alpha-1-antitrypsin deficiency	alpha-1-antitrypsin concentration

*More information can be found in subsequent chapters on the specific disease.

Radiological Procedures

Radiological tests may be used to evaluate patients with liver diseases. Each of these tests has certain strengths and all have limitations. The most common radiological procedures used in the evaluation of liver diseases are:

- Ultrasound or sonography
- Computerized axial tomography (CAT or CT) scan
- Magnetic resonance imaging (MRI) scan
- Liver-spleen scan
- Endoscopic retrograde cholangiopancreatography (ERCP)
- Tagged red blood cell scan

The methodology of performing them, the indications for, and the limitations of each of these tests are discussed below.

Ultrasound or Sonography

The ultrasound examination or sonogram is the most widely used radiological procedure to evaluate patients with liver diseases. The test is noninvasive and relatively cheap. To perform the test, "probes" that emit and detect sound waves are placed against the surface of the abdomen. An image based on the deflection and penetration of sound waves is then generated. There are virtually no risks to performing an ultrasound examination of the liver.

Ultrasound is an excellent test for the detection of liver masses such as tumors or cysts. It is also a very powerful method to determine widening of the bile ducts that can result from obstruction due to a stone or tumor. Ultrasound also provides a clear image of the gallbladder and is very sensitive for detecting gallstones. Combined with another type of sound wave analysis that detects Doppler shifts (a change in the pitch of a sound wave emanating or reflected from a moving object, such as the pitch of a train whistle when the train is moving toward or away from you), ultrasound can provide information about blood flow in the major veins and arteries of the liver.

Although often used on patients with acute and chronic hepatitis, an ultrasound provides very little to no useful information in such cases. Ultrasound cannot diagnose hepatitis (inflammation of the liver) or accurately assess the degree of inflammation or scar tissue (fibrosis) in the liver. Drug, alcoholic, or viral hepatitis cannot be diagnosed by ultrasound. Cirrhosis cannot be diagnosed reliably unless it is advanced and the liver is shrunken and nodular. The results of ultrasound scanning provide no information about liver function. Although an ultrasound can provide some clues as to the presence of fat in the liver, it is not by itself adequate to diagnose the condition known as fatty liver.

In sum, ultrasound is an excellent test for the detection of liver masses, assessment of bile ducts and gallbladder, and the detection of gallstones. It is not capable of assessing liver "function" or the degree of inflammation or fibrosis in hepatitis. It cannot diagnose cirrhosis unless it is advanced and the liver is shrunken or nodular. Ultrasound is noninvasive and there are no real risks associated with the procedure, except risks associated with additional testing due to inconclusive scans.

Computerized Axial Tomography (CAT or CT)

Computerized axial tomography, better known as CAT or CT scanning, generates an image based upon X-rays taken from multiple angles. To perform a CAT scan, the patient lies in a scanner shaped like a giant doughnut and X-rays are emitted and detected from multiple locations around the body. A computer reconstructs an image based upon the penetration and scattering of X-rays. CAT scan is a generally safe procedure with one of its few possible side effects being an allergic reaction to intravenous contrast dyes administered prior to the test. Intravenous contrast agents can also cause acute kidney failure in individuals with kidney problems.

CAT scanning of the liver has many of the same attributes as ultrasound. It is an excellent way to detect masses and gallstones and to image the gallbladder and bile ducts. It is one of the best tests to assess the extent of liver tumors and image the entire abdomen. It can also be used to accurately measure the size of the liver. CAT scans of the liver have most of the same limitations as ultrasound. Like ultrasound, CAT scans can diagnose cirrhosis only if it is advanced and the liver is shrunken and nodular. CAT scan cannot be used to diagnose hepatitis or estimate the degree of inflammation or scarring in the liver. CAT scans reveal nothing about liver function.

CAT scans are more expensive than ultrasound and more difficult to perform. It is not a routine test for individuals with liver diseases. In most cases, it should not be used in individuals with chronic liver disease unless tumors, other masses, bile duct disorders, or gallbladder disorders are suspected.

Magnetic Resonance Imaging (MRI)

Magnetic resonance imaging (MRI) uses nuclear magnetic resonance to produce images. The patient is placed in a very strong magnetic field to align the spins of the protons in the atoms in the patient's body. "Spin relaxation times" (spin relaxation time is the time it takes protons to change rotation when the body is pulsed with radio waves, which vary in different conditions) are measured and used to generate images of the internal organs. To perform a MRI scan, the patient is usually placed in a small "tunnel" that is surrounded by giant magnets. MRI is similar to CAT scan in its strengths and limitations. It may be slightly more sensitive for the evaluation of certain tumors.

Liver-Spleen Scan

The liver-spleen scan is a nuclear medicine test that can occasionally detect the presence of cirrhosis. In this test, a radioactive compound is injected into the patient and a picture taken with a camera that detects the emitted radiation. If blood flow to the liver is "backed up," as it could be in cirrhosis, the test will detect a "colloid shift" in which more of the radioactive material is taken up by the bone marrow as opposed to the liver. The liver-spleen scan is used less and less today and provides useful information only occasionally. It cannot diagnose cirrhosis in its early stages.

Tagged Red Blood Cell Scan

In a tagged red blood cell scan, a radioactive material is attached to red blood cells that are then injected into the patient's vein. A picture of the liver is taken with a camera that detects the emitted radioactivity. This test is excellent for one particular purpose: detection of hemangioma, a benign tumor of the liver. Because hemangioma has a very rich blood supply, the radioactive tagged red blood cells accumulate in it and the tumor is visualized by the camera.

Endoscopic Retrograde Cholangiopancreatography (ERCP)

ERCP is used to visualize the bile ducts and gallbladder. In ERCP, a fiber-optic tube (endoscope) is inserted into the patient's esophagus and passed to the small intestine. The patient is lightly sedated during this procedure. A smaller tube is then inserted into the end of the common bile duct that empties into the small intestine. Dye is injected into the bile duct to fill the smaller bile ducts within the liver and the ducts from the pancreas and gallbladder. After dye injection, X-ray images are taken of the upper abdomen. As the injected dye does not permit X-rays to pass through it, the filled structures appear white on a dark background. ERCP is the most sensitive procedure used to visualize the bile ducts. Subtle abnormalities or very small gallstones not seen on ultrasound or CT scanning can be detected. ERCP can also be modified to perform procedures such as removing gallstones stuck in the bile duct.

Liver Biopsy

Despite the availability of numerous blood tests and radiological procedures to assess the liver, biopsy provides critical information that none of the other tests can. In most chronic liver diseases, adequate diagnosis and treatment plans can be made only after a biopsy is performed. In short, in the absence of contraindications, liver biopsy is usually an important diagnostic test for all patients with chronic, but usually not acute, liver diseases.

Most liver biopsies are performed percutaneously (through the skin) with a needle. The patient is awake and not sedated. A percutaneous liver biopsy does not hurt that much. While the patient lies on his or her back, a spot in the right mid-axillary line (a line drawn roughly from the armpit to the hip) between two ribs is identified by the doctor (Figure 2.1). The area is cleaned with an antiseptic solution and numbed with lidocaine (similar to how the dentist numbs your mouth before filling a cavity). The doctor then breaks the tough surface skin with a

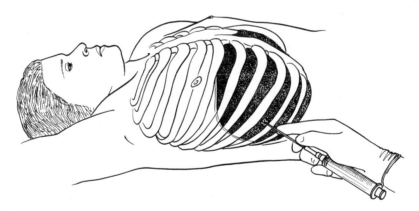

Figure 2.1. *Schematic diagram of how to perform a percutaneous needle biopsy of the liver.*

The patient lies on his back, and a spot in the right mid-axillary line between two ribs, as shown by the location of the needle in the diagram, is identified. The area is cleaned with an antiseptic solution and numbed with lidocaine. The doctor then breaks the tough surface skin with a sharp metal stick. A needle at the end of a syringe is then placed lightly into the small hole in the skin. While the patient is breathing calmly, the doctor rapidly sticks the needle into the liver and withdraws it in one swift motion that takes less than one second.

Illustration by Elizabeth Weadon Massari

sharp metal stick. A needle at the end of a syringe is then placed lightly into the small hole in the skin. While the patient is breathing calmly, the doctor rapidly sticks the needle into the liver and withdraws it in one swift motion that takes less than one second. In the process, a tiny piece of liver is sucked into the needle attached to the syringe. After the biopsy, the patient remains in bed for about four hours before being sent home. During this time, a nurse should periodically check the patient's pulse and blood pressure to ensure that there is no serious bleeding. I usually perform liver biopsies around 8 A.M. or 9 A.M., let the patient have lunch in bed around noon, and send him home around 1 P.M. or 2 P.M.

The thought of a liver biopsy often provokes considerable anxiety in the patient (and some doctors, too). However, if patients relax throughout the procedure, there is very little pain. The sensation associated with the actual biopsy (sticking a needle into the liver) has been described by many patients as feeling like being punched in the ribs. There may also be some dull pain in the right shoulder after the biopsy as irritation of the capsule of the liver is often referred as pain to that area. There is usually a little bleeding at the site of the biopsy but usually not more than can be routinely washed away with a couple of pieces of cotton.

In patients who do not have low platelet counts or elevated prothrombin times, percutaneous biopsy is a safe procedure. The major complication is bleeding that may very rarely require blood transfusion in less than 1 in 100 cases. Although deaths from percutaneous biopsy do occur, they are extremely rare in patients with normal platelet counts and prothrombin times who demonstrate absence of advanced liver disease, absence of fluid in the abdomen, or absence of bleeding disorders.

If the platelet count is too low, the prothrombin time too high, or significant ascites (fluid in the abdomen) is present, percutaneous liver biopsy should probably not be performed. In these cases, liver tissue can be obtained using other approaches. One alternative approach is to insert a catheter into the jugular vein in the neck. Another approach is through a laparoscope, an instrument inserted into the abdomen through which the doctor can see and cauterize bleeding areas. An open surgical liver biopsy can be performed as a last resort. Blind, percutaneous biopsy is also usually not appropriate if the aim is to obtain tissue from a liver tumor. In such cases, biopsy should be performed by a radiologist under ultrasound or CT guidance, with a laparoscope, or by a surgeon in an open procedure.

Why perform a liver biopsy? Several findings on biopsy are diagnostic for particular diseases. Others confirm the diagnosis suspected from clinical and laboratory data. Even if the diagnosis is relatively certain based on a patient's medical history, physical examination, and blood tests, however, a liver biopsy is usually the only way to know exactly what's going on in the liver. By looking at a piece of liver tissue under a microscope, the pathologist can determine the precise degree of inflammation in cases of chronic hepatitis. Biopsy can usually establish if chronic hepatitis is due to alcohol, viruses, or a combination of both. It is the only accurate way to diagnose fatty liver or hepatitis caused by fat. And unless cirrhosis is advanced, liver biopsy is the only way to establish its presence or absence.

Special studies can also be performed on liver tissue obtained at biopsy to definitively diagnose some diseases. For example, tissue iron content can be measured in suspected cases of familial hemochromatosis, in which case it would be elevated. Copper content can be measured in Wilson disease, in which case it will be high. Special tests can be performed on liver tissue and used to diagnose rare metabolic disorders such as glycogen storage diseases. Special stains of biopsy material can be used to detect accumulation of alpha-1-antitrypsin in cases of alpha-1-antitrypsin deficiency. Other special stains can be used to demonstrate the presence of viruses, other infectious agents, and certain types of cancer cells.

In sum, liver biopsy often provides data critical to the overall assessment of many patients with liver diseases. It is usually not necessary in acute liver diseases that resolve and in which a diagnosis can be established without it. In patients with chronic liver disease, however, liver biopsy is often the only way to clearly assess the status of the liver. It is also frequently the only way to determine the patient's prognosis, in particular the presence of cirrhosis.

The Failing Liver

Liver failure occurs when a large portion of hepatocytes die or cease to function. The liver can fail with sudden or acute loss of liver cell function in an otherwise healthy body. The presentation in such cases of sudden liver failure is dramatic. Liver failure can also occur gradually in patients with cirrhosis who slowly lose liver function over time. Patients with cirrhosis can also suddenly suffer from liver failure as a result of a new insult to an organ that is functioning only marginally.

As with liver diseases in general, liver failure can be broken down into two categories: acute and chronic. Although many signs and symptoms overlap, there are important differences. The first part of this chapter will focus on acute or sudden liver failure in individuals who do not have underlying liver disease. In particular, it will focus on the most severe type of acute liver failure which is known as *fulminant hepatic failure*. The second part of this chapter will focus on chronic liver failure, which in virtually all cases occurs as a result of cirrhosis. Some complications from cirrhosis, however, do not result from loss of hepatocytes per se, but from abnormal architecture of the cirrhotic liver.

Fulminant Hepatic Failure

Fulminant hepatic failure is acute liver failure with hepatic encephalopathy. Hepatic encephalopathy is abnormal mental functioning that results from failure of the liver to remove ammonia and other toxins from the blood. Several investigators have proposed slightly different definitions for fulminant hepatic failure. Common to all of these definitions is the acute onset of liver failure with hepatic encephalopathy. The term *fulminant hepatic failure* should not be used for patients with underlying chronic liver disease. In fulminant hepatic failure, encephalopathy must result directly from, and occur concurrently or within, a short time after the acute liver injury. The term *fulminant hepatic failure* should not be used unless liver failure is acute and accompanied by encephalopathy. If encephalopathy is not present but other signs and symptoms of liver dysfunction are, the condition should be described as acute liver failure.

The patient with fulminant hepatic failure will have other indications of liver failure besides hepatic encephalopathy. These usually include jaundice and may, after some time, include ascites and edema. Blood ALT and AST activities will often be markedly elevated as a result of the massive hepatocyte necrosis that causes fulminant hepatic failure. Blood AST and ALT activities may be elevated for only a few days, however, and then rapidly return to normal or near normal. Remember, ALT and

AST activities are *not* liver function tests. Right after an acute, massive injury to the liver, the blood ALT and AST activities will be extremely high—even thousands of times above normal—because all of the liver hepatocytes die suddenly. Blood AST and ALT activities will then return to normal in a few days as virtually no more hepatocytes remain to die. Despite having normal aminotransferase activities at this time, a patient's liver may not be functioning.

Fulminant hepatic failure is almost always associated with elevated bilirubin concentration in the blood and prolonged prothrombin time. When hepatocytes die, bilirubin is no longer metabolized sufficiently in the liver and the serum concentration rises. As the conjugating ability of the liver is very high, the few remaining hepatocytes may conjugate bilirubin but it will not be secreted into bile and return into the blood. As a result, both direct and, to some extent, indirect bilirubin concentrations in the blood can rise in fulminant hepatic failure. Similarly, production of clotting factors normally made in hepatocytes is reduced significantly and prothrombin time increases. In fact, the degree of prolongation of prothrombin time is a fairly good predictor of the severity of liver failure. If liver function does not return to normal, then albumin concentration in the blood will also begin to fall over a period of several days to weeks as its synthesis also decreases.

In fulminant hepatic failure, encephalopathy can progress to coma if liver function does not return. Brain edema or swelling can also result from fulminant hepatic failure that can lead to irreversible brain damage and death. The kidneys and lungs may also fail and the patient becomes susceptible to massive infections. Bleeding complications occur because clotting factors are no longer adequately synthesized and the platelet count gradually falls.

Causes of Fulminant Hepatic Failure

Many of the agents that cause acute liver disease can cause fulminant hepatic failure. In addition, shock caused by hemorrhage, severe dehydration, heatstroke, or overwhelming infection (sepsis) can cause the liver to fail. In many patients admitted to hospitals with fulminant hepatic failure, the cause is never determined. This may be because the patient deteriorates too rapidly or is too sick for appropriate diagnostic tests to be performed. Sometimes the cause, such as ingestion of a toxin, is never witnessed or reported by the patient. Table 3.1 lists some of the causes of fulminant hepatic failure.

Wilson disease and autoimmune hepatitis are included the list in Table 3.1 in quotation marks. Individuals with these diseases can present with sudden onset liver failure with encephalopathy that appears identical to fulminant hepatic failure. These diseases are chronic but can present as acute liver failure. Therefore, precisely speaking, the term *fulminant hepatic failure* does not apply in a patient with a chronic liver disease, even if the disease presents as sudden liver failure with encephalopathy.

Treatment

Patients with fulminant hepatic failure are among the sickest in any hospital. The major goal of treatment is to keep the patient alive and free of serious complications until liver function spontaneously recovers or emergency liver transplantation can be performed. In some patients, hepatocytes regenerate and liver function returns to normal. Until liver function returns, however, the patient may be comatose and suffer from numerous complications. In other cases, liver function never returns and the patient dies unless liver transplantation is performed. One of the major challenges in caring for patients with fulminant

Table 3.1. *Some causes of fulminant hepatic failure.*

Wilson disease and autoimmune hepatitis are listed in quotation marks because, although patients with these disorders can present with signs and symptoms identical to fulminant hepatic failure, both are technically chronic diseases.

Acute viral hepatitis	Hepatitis A
	Hepatitis B
	Hepatitis C (rarely)
	Hepatitis D
	Hepatitis E
	Yellow fever
	Others (very rare)
Drugs and toxins	Overdose of acetaminophen (over-the-counter pain reliever)
	Halothane (rarely used)
	Isoniazid (used to treat tuberculosis)
	Amanita phalloides (poisonous mushrooms)
	Carbon tetrachloride
	Others
"Shock liver"	Hemorrhage
	Sepsis (overwhelming infection)
	Heatstroke
	Heart failure
	Severe dehydration
Other causes	Fatty liver of pregnancy
	"Wilson disease"
	"Autoimmune hepatitis"

hepatic failure is to try to predict in which cases liver function will return with supportive care only, and in which instances emergency liver transplantation will be absolutely necessary to save the patient's life. This is not always easy.

Patients with fulminant hepatic failure should be admitted to an intensive care unit. Treatment is directed at support, prevention, and dealing with complications. Patients must often be put on ventilators to assist with breathing, and dialysis may be necessary if kidney failure occurs. Intravenous fluid support is required and antibiotics are frequently necessary to fight infections. Transfusions of blood and blood products are often required to treat bleeding complications. If the patient goes into a deep coma, a monitor to measure central nervous system pressure is inserted through the skull. The pressure in the patient's brain is carefully monitored because a sudden increase in brain swelling can lead to rapid death. If significant brain swelling occurs, rapid liver transplantation may be needed to prevent death. Once brain swelling becomes severe, nothing can be done to save the patient.

A patient with fulminant hepatic failure should ideally be transferred to a center where liver transplantation can be performed. Doctors at transplant centers have the most experience in determining which patients will not recover and which ones will require liver transplantation to survive. Liver transplantation can be done only at these medical centers.

Cirrhosis and Its Complications

Many people associate cirrhosis only with excessive alcohol consumption. Although alcohol is the leading cause of cirrhosis in the U.S., it can be caused by virtually any chronic liver disease. Cirrhosis is characterized anatomically by widespread nodules in the liver and fibrosis. Fibrosis is the deposition of scar tissue that results from ongoing inflammation and liver cell death. Nodules form as dying liver cells are replaced by regenerating cells. Unfortunately, this regeneration results in abnormal liver architecture.

Cirrhosis can be clinically inapparent. In its early stages, the nodules and fibrosis of cirrhosis may be detected only by examination of tissue obtained by liver biopsy. The patient may have no symptoms and live a normal, sometimes very active life. Ultimately, the fibrosis and nodule formation in cirrhosis can cause distortion of the liver architecture that interferes with blood flow through the organ. Cirrhosis can also lead to an inability of the liver to perform its biochemical functions. As cirrhosis becomes advanced, the abnormalities in the liver's blood flow and biochemical functions lead to several potentially serious complications such as:

- Splenomegaly (enlarged spleen)
- Bleeding from esophageal and gastric varices (varicose veins)
- Edema (generalized fluid retention)
- Ascites (fluid retention, specifically in abdomen)
- Jaundice (yellow discoloration of skin from bilirubin retention)
- Encephalopathy (mental changes from mild confusion to coma)
- Bleeding tendencies
- Low or high blood sugars
- Increased susceptibility to infections
- Spontaneous bacterial peritonitis (infected fluid in abdomen)

- Kidney failure
- Generalized muscle wasting
- Hyponatremia (low blood sodium concentration)

Portal Hypertension

In cirrhosis, blood flow through the liver is impeded because of the abnormal architecture. As a result, blood backs up in the portal vein and portal circulation. This leads to elevated blood pressure in the portal circulation which is known as *portal hypertension*. Portal hypertension can also sometimes occur in severe cases of acute hepatitis and other forms of liver damage. Cirrhosis is by far the leading cause, however. Portal hypertension can cause several serious problems:

- *Splenomegaly*—Because the portal vein is connected to the splenic vein, portal hypertension can cause blood to back up in the spleen. This causes the spleen to become enlarged (splenomegaly) and trap blood cells. Sequestration of platelets in an abnormally enlarged spleen can cause a drop in the platelet count and abnormal bleeding tendencies.
- *Esophageal and gastric varices*—As the pressure in the portal circulation increases, blood can flow backward from the portal circulation into the systemic venous circulation at certain points where they are connected. Prominent connections between the portal and systemic venous circulations occur in the esophagus and stomach. Portal hypertension can therefore lead to varicose veins in the stomach and esophagus. Varicose veins in the stomach and esophagus are known as gastric and esophageal *varices,* respectively. Portal and systemic circulations are also connected in the rectum and increased portal pres-

sure can cause hemorrhoids. The two circulations also connect under the skin on the abdomen and increased pressure can cause prominent visible veins and a swollen collection of congested veins known as a *caput medusa.*

Gastric and esophageal varices are one of the most serious complications of portal hypertension because they can rupture and bleed. Internal bleeding from esophageal and gastric varices can be massive and life threatening. The patient will often experience nausea and vomiting when gastric or esophageal varices bleed. The vomitus usually has a "coffee grounds" appearance that results from the action of stomach acid on blood, which causes clumps of normally soluble material to denature and fall out of solution. As a result, the blood looks like coffee grounds. Bleeding gastric or esophageal varices can also cause black, tarry stools, known as *melana,* if partially digested blood passes through the digestive tract. Patients with either coffee grounds *emesis* (vomit) or melana (black stools) should head immediately to the emergency room, as these symptoms are usually a result of brisk internal bleeding into the upper gastrointestinal tract.

- *Ascites and edema*—Hypertension in the portal circulation, along with complex hormonal, metabolic, and possibly kidney abnormalities in cirrhosis, can lead to fluid accumulation. *Edema* is the general term for fluid retention in the body. In cirrhosis, there is a tendency for fluid to be retained in the abdomen. This is termed *ascites.* In cirrhosis, ascites may not be present or may be massive (gallons of fluid). It is not uncommon for a patient with cirrhosis to first seek medical attention because he or she can no longer fit into a dress or pair of pants. Because of the tendency to retain fluid, patients with cirrhosis should have their weight checked periodically.

Jaundice

Bilirubin is taken up by the healthy liver, conjugated to a more water-soluble form, and secreted into the bile (see chapter 1). In cirrhosis, there is decreased bilirubin secretion from hepatocytes. This leads to backup of bilirubin in the blood, elevated blood bilirubin concentrations (usually mostly direct bilirubin, see chapter 2), and jaundice. As the conjugated form of bilirubin backs up, bilirubin can spill into the urine, giving it a bright yellow to dark brown color.

Hepatic Encephalopathy

Hepatic encephalopathy is abnormal brain function that can range from subtle mental status changes to deep coma. Hepatic encephalopathy occurs in both fulminant hepatic failure (see above) and advanced cirrhosis. In cirrhosis, some toxin-laden blood leaving the gut bypasses the liver hepatocytes as a result of the abnormal architecture. Metabolism of certain toxic compounds absorbed in the gut may also be decreased within the liver as biochemical function deteriorates. Both of these derangements can lead to hepatic encephalopathy as toxic metabolites, normally removed from the blood by the liver, reach the brain.

In its early stages, hepatic encephalopathy is characterized by subtle mental changes such as poor concentration or irritability. One of the first problems in hepatic encephalopathy is the inability to construct simple objects such as a six-point star out of toothpicks. Various degrees of confusion and sleepiness occur in more advanced cases. In severe cases, hepatic encephalopathy is manifested as stupor or coma.

Infectious Complications

Individuals with cirrhosis may have depressed immune systems and are at higher risk for more types of infections than healthy individuals. One infectious complication unique to individuals with ascites is *spontaneous bacterial peritonitis* or *SBP*. In SBP, the abnormally retained fluid in the abdomen becomes spontaneously infected by the bacteria present in the colon. If not adequately treated with antibiotics, SBP can lead to sepsis, an overwhelming infection of the blood.

Other Complications

Cachexia

Patients with cirrhosis have generalized wasting, which is known as cachexia. In advanced cirrhosis, there is significant loss of muscle mass even if nutrient intake is maintained. This is usually most noticeable in the temporal muscles on the sides of head just in front of the ears. Patients with end-stage cirrhosis and ascites often look like balloons with toothpicks for arms and legs as fluid accumulates in the abdomen and muscle mass is lost in the extremities.

It is not entirely understood why muscle wasting occurs in patients with cirrhosis or other chronic diseases. It may result, in part, from the abnormal secretion of various cytokines (compounds secreted into the blood that alter body metabolism). As a result, patients develop an overall metabolic state in which muscle proteins are degraded more rapidly than they are synthesized. Patients with cirrhosis usually have high circulating levels of the cytokine tumor necrosis factor, which is also known as cachexia because it causes wasting when injected into animals.

Bleeding tendencies

In cirrhosis, the platelet counts fall secondary to abnormal trapping of platelets in an enlarged spleen. The prothrombin time is also increased as a result of decreased synthesis of certain blood clotting factors in the failing liver. As a result of both of these alterations, individuals with cirrhosis have an increased chance of bleeding. Decreased blood clotting capability can be a major aggravating factor in patients with gastric or esophageal varices that rupture and bleed. The odds of stopping the bleeding lessen as well.

Electrolyte abnormalities

Abnormalities in total body fluid balance and altered kidney and hormone function in cirrhosis can lead to problems with blood *electrolytes*. Electrolytes are soluble elements in the form of ions in the blood. The most abundant electrolytes in the blood are sodium and chloride (table salt). Bicarbonate and potassium are also important blood electrolytes. Significant abnormalities in their concentrations can result in numerous problems.

The electrolyte abnormality most often seen in advanced cirrhosis, especially in patients with edema and ascites, is *hyponatremia* or an abnormally low blood sodium concentration. Severe hyponatremia (very low blood sodium concentrations) can cause seizures and other brain abnormalities. Although sodium concentration in the blood may be low, total body sodium paradoxically increases in patients with cirrhosis and hyponatremia. Administration of excess sodium only worsens the problem by increasing the amount of ascites and edema. Because patients with cirrhosis and ascites may have subtle kidney abnormalities and are often thirsty secondary to hormonal changes, drinking of excess water contributes to hyponatremia. Therefore, hyponatremia will generally improve with restriction of free water intake. In very severe cases of hyponatremia, intravenous administration of concentrated sodium solutions may be necessary to prevent seizures, even though this may worsen ascites and edema. This must be done slowly and carefully.

Kidney abnormalities

Cirrhosis also leads to abnormalities in kidney function that range from mild to complete kidney shutdown. Subtle alterations in kidney function and consequent hormonal changes contribute to the formation of ascites and edema and the development of hyponatremia. In advanced cases of cirrhosis, a type of kidney failure known as *hepatorenal syndrome* can occur. In hepatorenal syndrome, the kidneys fail to function in the cirrhotic body for reasons that are unclear. Surprisingly, the same kidneys work fine if they are put in a normal body. Therefore, there is something about advanced cirrhosis that makes them shut down. Hepatorenal syndrome can be treated with dialysis for a short time; however, it is virtually always fatal unless liver transplantation is performed. When the liver is replaced in a patient with hepatorenal syndrome, kidney function returns to normal.

Other metabolic complications

There are several other metabolic complications associated with cirrhosis including:
- Low blood albumin concentration, which can enhance formation of ascites and edema.
- The metabolism of many drugs is decreased and the dosages of some medications must be adjusted appropriately.
- In men, breast enlargement or *gynecomastia* sometimes occurs because metabolism of estrogens by the liver is decreased. Atrophy of the testicles can also occur.

- Derangements in the metabolism of triglycerides and cholesterol can occur. Blood cholesterol concentration is usually very low, except in cases of cirrhosis caused by bile duct obstruction where it can be abnormally elevated.
- Abnormalities in sugar metabolism including, in earlier stages, insulin resistance that leads to high blood sugars. In advanced stages of cirrhosis, however, blood sugar may be dangerously low because it cannot be synthesized from glycogen, fats, or proteins in the failing liver.

Diagnosis of Cirrhosis

Cirrhosis is usually an easy diagnosis when some or all of the above complications are present in a chronically ill individual with a history of liver disease. Virtually any chronic liver disease can cause cirrhosis. The underlying cause of cirrhosis can be identified in most cases though sometimes it remains elusive. Such cases are called "cryptogenic" cirrhosis, which is not really a diagnosis but a term signifying that the disease that caused cirrhosis cannot be determined. Conditions such as metastatic cancer, clots in the hepatic or portal veins, severe acute hepatitis, or acute bile duct obstruction can cause some of the same abnormalities observed in patients with cirrhosis. A careful history, combined with special diagnostic tests, will usually identify these conditions.

As emphasized in previous chapters, some individuals with cirrhosis, especially early in the course of the disease, will have no overt clinical signs or symptoms. Radiological and nuclear medicine tests suggest the presence of cirrhosis in only a few of these cases. In most patients without clinical complications, a diagnosis of cirrhosis usually requires liver biopsy (see chapter 2).

Treatment of the Patient with Cirrhosis

Cirrhosis of the liver is irreversible. Scarring and nodules cannot revert to normal liver architecture. Treatment of the underlying liver disease may slow or stop the progression of cirrhosis, i.e., the laying down of additional scar tissue and formation of new nodules. This may prevent the development of complications and serious liver dysfunction. For example, termination of alcohol intake may stop the progression of alcoholic cirrhosis. Treatment of metabolic liver diseases may also slow the progression of cirrhosis. Chronic viral hepatitis B and C may respond to treatment with interferon or other medications and autoimmune hepatitis may improve with immunosuppressive drugs.

Most "treatments" in patients with cirrhosis are directed at reversing or preventing complications (Table 3.2). When cirrhosis is advanced, some complications become nearly impossible to treat or prevent. This condition is commonly referred to as "end-stage" liver disease. In so-called end-stage liver disease, transplantation is the only option. Hence, careful periodic follow-up by a doctor knowledgeable in liver diseases is an important aspect in the care of patients with cirrhosis. If the complications of cirrhosis become uncontrollable, or when an experienced physician realizes that they will soon become uncontrollable, referral to a liver transplantation center is essential. Fortunately, in many cases, complications of cirrhosis respond to the various interventions described below.

Bleeding from esophageal or gastric varices

Bleeding from esophageal or gastric varices is treated immediately using intravenous fluids and blood transfusions as necessary. Fluid and blood should be given immediately if the patient is not stable. The diagnosis is generally made by *endoscopy,*

Table 3.2. *Treatments for some complications of cirrhosis.*

Bleeding from esophageal varices	Endoscopic sclerotherapy
	Endoscopic rubber band ligation
	Beta-blockers and possibly nitrates
	Vasopressin and somatostatin analogue (emergencies only)
	Balloon compression (emergencies only)
	Transjugular intrahepatic portosystemic shunt (TIPS)
	Surgical portal-systemic shunts
Edema and ascites	Low sodium diet (very important)
	Diuretics (spironolactone usually first choice)
	Paracentesis (removal of ascites with needle)
Encephalopathy	Low protein diet
	Lactulose
	Neomycin
Bleeding tendencies	Vitamin K
	Fresh frozen plasma (emergencies only)
Spontaneous bacterial peritonitis	Antibiotics
Hyponatremia (low blood sodium concentration)	Restriction of free water intake

giving the doctor a direct view of the bleeding varices (or other possible sources of bleeding).

If bleeding esophageal varices are identified, sclerotherapy or rubber band ligation are usually first-line treatments. Both of these procedures are done through the endoscope. Sclerotherapy is accomplished by injection of a caustic substance into the varicose vein. In rubber band ligation, rubber bands are ligated (tied) around varices to stop bleeding and obliterate them. Gastric varices cannot be treated by sclerotherapy because the caustic chemical can irritate the stomach and cause it to rupture. Gastric varices can sometimes be treated by rubber band ligation.

Sclerotherapy or rubber band ligation should be performed only on patients who have varices that are actively bleeding or have been previously documented to bleed. If varices are detected incidentally but have never bled, these treatments are not indicated. If sclerotherapy or rubber band ligation stops variceal bleeding, follow-up endoscopy should be performed on a regular schedule and repeat courses of sclerotherapy or rubber band ligation should be performed until all visible esophageal varices are obliterated.

Beta-blockers and nitrates are oral drugs used to prevent bleeding. Several studies have shown that these medications can decrease the incidence of bleeding or re-bleeding from esophageal varices. Once acute bleeding is stopped, or if varices are incidentally found that have not yet bled, beta-blockers and nitrates are often prescribed.

Sometimes, endoscopic sclerotherapy or rubber band ligation cannot stop acute bleeding from esophageal or gastric varices. In other cases, bleeding may result from a condition known as portal gastropathy in which the pressure is increased diffusely in the veins of the stomach but there is no single prominent varicose vein to ligate. In this case, the patient should be admitted to an intensive care unit where medical therapy with vasopression or somatostatin may be attempted. These medications constrict some blood vessels and/or lower portal pressures.

If acute bleeding from esophageal varices does not stop despite attempted endoscopic and medical treatment, balloon compression may be used as a lifesaving option. A tube with a large balloon at the end is inserted into the esophagus and the balloon is then inflated. The inflated balloon may stop bleeding by direct compression.

Shunts are surgical connections that are made between the portal circulation—which has increased pressure in cirrhosis—and the systemic circulation. Shunts can stop bleeding from gastric or esophageal varices in individuals with cirrhosis and portal hypertension because they lower the blood pressure in the portal system. In classical open surgical shunt procedures, a major vein of the portal circulation is directly connected to a major vein of the lower pressure systemic circulation. For example, the portal vein may be connected directly to the vena cava, or the splenic vein (which is connected to the portal vein) to a vein leading to a kidney. These connections allow some portal blood to bypass the cirrhotic liver, causing pressure in the portal system to be lower. The major complication of surgical shunts is worsening of hepatic encephalopathy as a larger portion of portal blood bypasses the liver and cannot be detoxified.

Surgical shunt procedures are rarely performed today. More recently, a less invasive shunt procedure has been developed and is generally performed by radiologists. This procedure is known as *transjugular intrahepatic portosystemic shunt* or TIPS. In TIPS, a hollow tube is placed directly into the liver from an approach through the jugular vein in the neck. The tube is placed to connect the portal vein and hepatic vein directly through the liver thus allowing some of the blood to bypass the cirrhotic architecture and relieve pressure in the portal circulation. Patients undergoing TIPS are also at increased risk for developing worsening hepatic encephalopathy afterward. In addition, the shunt may clot with time, again increasing the risk of bleeding from gastric or esophageal varices. Despite these complications, TIPS can be lifesaving.

Edema and ascites

The most important initial therapeutic intervention to prevent ascites and edema in cirrhosis is a strict, low-salt diet. In individuals with significant ascites and/or edema, a daily allowance of only 500 mg of sodium chloride is ideal; however, most patients find this kind of diet terribly unpalatable. Nonetheless, it is important that the patient do everything possible to significantly restrict salt consumption. Virtually all canned and processed foods should be avoided at all costs. Meat and fish should be consumed only in small quantities as these foods contain significant amounts of salt. A patient with cirrhosis and ascites should (generally) stick to a mostly vegetarian diet with low-salt fruits, grains, pastas, and vegetables providing most of the calories. An occasional egg and infrequent, small portions of meat, but no cured or processed meats such as salami or pastrami, may be consumed. The bottom line is that the patient's diet should be as salt-free as possible with every effort necessary to reduce the intake of foods, including meats, that contain high salt content. If a cirrhotic patient with ascites and edema also has hyponatremia (low blood sodium concentration), free water intake should also be restricted. Water is restricted to usually one quart per day or less until blood sodium concentrations return to near normal.

If diet alone does not control edema and ascites, the next step is to add a diuretic. Diuretics are not substitutes for a low-salt diet but are complementary. The first choice diuretic is usually spironolactone (Aldactone®). Spironolactone works by countering the effects of aldosterone, a hormone that acts on kidneys whose blood levels are abnormally increased in cirrhotic individuals with ascites and edema. If spironolactone and diet do not control ascites and edema, a second diuretic medication with a different mechanism of action is cautiously added. Either hydrochlorothiazide, or a so-called "loop diuretic" such as furosemide (Lasix®), is added next. Patients with cirrhosis who are taking diuretics should be followed closely by their doctors to monitor (possible) excessive intravascular dehydration, and their kidney function should be checked periodically.

If diet and diuretics do not relieve ascites and abdominal swelling becomes so intense that it is painful, or the patient has difficulty breathing due to compression on the diaphragm, large-volume *paracentesis* is an option. In this procedure, a needle is inserted into the abdomen through the skin and fluid is drained gradually. About four to six liters (one liter is approximately one quart) can be drained at a time. Sometimes, an infusion of albumin will be given at the time paracentesis is performed. In some patients with advanced cirrhosis, repeated large-volume paracenteses are required.

A type of surgical procedure is available in refractory ascites that cannot be managed by recurrent large-volume paracentesis treatments. This procedure is associated with serious complications and is used very rarely these days as repeated large-volume paracentesis can usually be employed to treat a patient until liver transplantation can be performed. The surgical procedure, known as a Denver or a Laveen shunt, places a tube with a one-way valve between the intra-abdominal space and a large vein. As a result of this shunting, the ascites fluid drains directly into the patient's bloodstream. Although theoretically appealing, serious complications such as infection, clotting of the shunt, and disseminated intravascular coagulation (abnormal clotting of the blood), are common after this procedure. Denver or Laveen shunts are usually reserved as last-resort comfort measures for individuals who have massive ascites and are not eligible for liver transplantation.

Spontaneous bacterial peritonitis

Patients with ascites are at risk for spontaneous bacterial peritonitis. This infection should be considered in any patient with ascites who develops fever or abdominal pain. Sometimes, spontaneous bacterial peritonitis will present as a general deterioration in overall condition or worsening hepatic encephalopathy in the absence of fever. The diagnostic procedure for spontaneous bacterial peritonitis is *paracentesis*. Usually, only a small volume of ascites fluid needs to be removed with a needle and syringe. The diagnosis of spontaneous bacterial peritonitis is made if the white blood cell count in the ascites fluid is elevated. Treatment with antibiotics is essential and usually done intravenously in the hospital. Some studies have suggested that long-term oral antibiotics may be useful to prevent subsequent infections in individuals with recurrent episodes of spontaneous bacterial peritonitis.

Hepatic encephalopathy

First step in the treatment of hepatic encephalopathy is a low-protein diet. Proteins are high in nitrogen content. Ammonia and other nitrogen-containing compounds, which are toxic to the brain when not removed by the cirrhotic liver, are produced by the metabolism of proteins by bacteria in the colon. Therefore, meats, nuts, and other high protein foods should be consumed only in very low quantities by individuals with hepatic encephalopathy. Vegetables, fruits, grains, and pastas should be substituted. The diet is in many aspects similar to the low-salt diet for ascites and edema.

The first-line drug treatment is usually lactulose. Lactulose is a sugar that is not absorbed from the gut. In part, it acts as a laxative to expel nitrogen-containing compounds from the colon before bacteria can metabolize them into substances toxic to an individual with a liver that cannot adequately clear them from the blood. Lactulose also causes the inside of the gut to be increasingly acidic, making it less favorable for nitrogen-containing toxins and ammonia to be absorbed. Another drug treatment for encephalopathy is neomycin, an antibiotic not absorbed from the gut which kills bacteria in the colon that produce ammonia and other nitrogen-containing toxic compounds.

Bleeding tendencies

Administration of vitamin K can sometimes help the decreased production of clotting factors in patients with cirrhosis. In emergency bleeding situations, or prior to invasive medical procedures that may be necessary, fresh frozen plasma can be transfused intravenously. Fresh frozen plasma is the component of blood from which red and white cells have been removed; it contains clotting factors and other proteins. Platelet transfusions may also be given to patients with low platelet counts to help stop or prevent bleeding.

Liver transplantation

In some patients, the complications of cirrhosis become refractory to all medical therapies. As the liver continues to fail, hepatic encephalopathy worsens, ascites continues to accumulate, and other complications worsen. These complications may no longer be responsive to medical interventions. Cachexia and muscle wasting cannot be halted no matter how many nutrients the patient receives. Kidney function may gradually fail and hepatorenal syndrome (see above) may develop. In these advanced cases of cirrhosis—also known as end-stage liver disease—only liver transplantation can save the patient's life. The general goal of liver transplantation is to replace the patient's liver just before complications of cirrhosis become refractory to medical treatment. In ideal cases, this can be estimated. In many cases, however, there is considerable uncertainty as to how soon the complications of cirrhosis and liver failure will become life-threatening. Patients with cirrhosis and one or more of its complications should probably be evaluated at a center for liver transplantation at least two years before the doctor anticipates that the condition will deteriorate and medical treatment will no longer suffice to control the complications. Liver transplantation is discussed in more detail in chapter 5.

CHAPTER 4

Diseases of the Liver

Previous chapters addressed the functions of the normal liver and what can go wrong, in general, in liver diseases. The most serious consequences of liver disease, fulminant hepatic failure and cirrhosis, were also addressed. This chapter covers specific diseases that affect the liver and, in some cases, can cause cirrhosis and liver failure.

Alcoholic Liver Disease

Most people readily recognize ethyl alcohol as a major cause of liver disease. In the U.S., alcohol is the number one cause of liver disease. Although it has been estimated that as many as 10 percent of Americans abuse alcohol, most people who drink excessively do not develop liver disease. It is not known why some

individuals who regularly have only a few drinks per day will develop liver disease, while others who drink a bottle or more of
hard liquor a day will not. What is important to realize is that
excessive alcohol consumption can potentially cause liver disease
in an individual, and it is not possible to predict in whom this
will happen. Anyone who consumes too much alcohol on a regular basis is at risk to develop liver disease.

Alcoholic liver disease presents in many different ways. Some
examples may help illustrate the many different signs and symptoms:

CASE 1. A thirty-five-year-old homeless man is brought to the
emergency room by a city Emergency Medical Services ambulance after being found lying in the street confused and agi-
tated. He is dirty, disheveled, and looks much older than his
actual age. He has a fever, is deeply jaundiced, and is breathing
rapidly. Laboratory examination reveals elevated blood ALT
and AST activities with the AST activity being almost three
times higher. Bilirubin is elevated, albumin is low, and prothrombin time is prolonged. Chest X-ray indicates pneumonia
and many old fractured ribs. The medical resident who admits
the patient recognizes him as someone who is always seen on
the street near her apartment with a bottle of hard liquor or
fortified wine. He is hospitalized and treated with antibiotics
but becomes tremulous, suffers a seizure, and remains critically
ill for about a week. He is treated with benzodiazepines. After
several weeks in the hospital, his condition gradually improves.
Upon discharge, he is no longer jaundiced and ALT and AST
activities are near normal, though blood albumin concentration
is still a little low. He refuses referral to an inpatient rehabilitation center, and the medical resident who admitted the patient
sees him on the street with a bottle of fortified wine a few days
after discharge.

CASE 2. A fifty-two-year-old woman is the mother of two grown children and wife of a CEO of a large multinational corporation. Her children no longer live at home and her husband, who travels frequently, is now seeking a divorce. She has been arrested twice in the past year for driving her BMW while under the influence of alcohol. After considerable urging by her daughter, she sees her family doctor. She denies having more than a few drinks a week, but blood tests indicate numerous abnormalities, including elevated serum ALT and AST activities, elevated GGTP activity, and slightly low albumin concentration. She is referred to a liver specialist who performs a liver biopsy. Cirrhosis is confirmed.

CASE 3. A twenty-year-old student at an Ivy league college starts drinking heavily for the first time in his life. After a few months, he is consuming at least twelve beers a night plus hard liquor. He goes to the student emergency health services facility because of nausea and vomiting mixed with red blood. Blood tests show mildly elevated ALT, AST, and GGTP activities; a complete blood count reveals mildly elevated mean corpuscular volume (slightly enlarged red blood cells). He is admitted to the local hospital. An upper endoscopy indicates a tear in his esophagus (Mallory-Weiss tear) that was bleeding, and he is discharged. He attends a campus support group for students with alcohol problems, gives up drinking, and starts exercising regularly. On follow-up examination a few months later, he is in excellent health and a laboratory examination is completely normal.

One theme central to these three hypothetical cases of alcoholic liver disease, and all real cases, is excessive alcohol intake. Alcoholic liver disease is virtually always associated with the psychiatric diagnoses that are known as alcohol use disorders. Most people refer to these conditions as "alcoholism" and individuals that suffer from them as "alcoholics." Therefore, before discussing the effects of alcohol on the liver, it is essential to understand something about misuse of alcohol.

"Alcoholism"

"Alcoholism" is an ill-defined term for the condition characterized by alcohol consumption that causes psychosocial or medical problems. Everyone would recognize the patient in case 1 above as the typical "skid row alcoholic" but may have a harder time recognizing the patients in cases 2 and 3 as having disorders caused by alcohol until it is too late. In fact, an alcohol use disorder was recognized too late in case 2. Fortunately for the patient described in case 3, he had a problem that brought him to medical attention early in life.

Like "alcoholism," the adjective "alcoholic" is an imprecise term used to describe an individual who has psychosocial or medical problems resulting from excessive alcohol consumption. The *Diagnostic and Statistical Manual of Mental Disorders, Fourth Edition,* of the American Psychiatric Association provides specific diagnostic criteria for two chronic alcohol use disorders: *alcohol dependence* and *alcohol abuse.* The less precise term "alcoholic" would include individuals with either of these conditions. Although it is not precise, I will sometimes use the term "alcoholic" in this book.

The clinical criteria for alcohol abuse are maladaptive patterns of use leading to clinically significant impairment or distress occurring within a twelve-month period. This basically means persistent and serious social and personal problems that result from drinking alcohol. An example would be failure to perform adequately at work, in school, or at home as a result of being drunk or hung over. Another example would be the use of alcohol in physically hazardous situations, such as driving a car or operating machinery while intoxicated. Individuals with alcohol abuse disorders may experience other substance-related social problems, such as arrests for disorderly conduct or fighting while intoxicated. More importantly, people with alcohol abuse disorders will continue to drink despite having the types of problems that are caused or exacerbated by consuming alcohol. To have a diagnosis of substance abuse, the individual must have never met the criteria for substance dependence.

Two central features of alcohol dependence are *tolerance* and *withdrawal*. Tolerance is characterized by a need for increased amounts of alcohol to achieve intoxication or diminished effects with continued use of the same amount of a substance. Withdrawal is a constellation of signs and symptoms that occur if a dependent individual suddenly stops drinking alcohol (see below). Other criteria for alcohol dependence include consumption in larger amounts or over longer periods than intended, persistent desire or unsuccessful efforts to reduce consumption, and spending a great deal of time in activities necessary to obtain it. Individuals with alcohol dependence may also reduce important social, occupational, or recreational activities because of alcohol use. An important aspect of alcohol dependence, especially concerning the patient with alcoholic liver disease, is continued use of alcohol despite knowledge of having a physical or psychological problem caused or exacerbated by it. In other words, an individual with liver disease related to alcohol who continues to drink, despite knowing that it is harmful, has already met one of the criteria for alcohol dependence.

Alcohol withdrawal is a characteristic syndrome that occurs when a dependent individual stops or reduces alcohol intake that has been heavy and prolonged. The hypothetical patient in case 1 above suffered from alcohol withdrawal after admission to the hospital. The syndrome of alcohol withdrawal includes tremor, insomnia, sweating, rapid pulse rate, nausea, vomiting, psychomotor agitation, and anxiety. Alcohol withdrawal can also cause hallucinations and delusions, one common hallucination being that bugs are crawling over the individual's body (this is known as formication). The syndrome of alcohol withdrawal is sometimes called *delirium tremens* or *DTs* because delirium and tremulousness are characteristic symptoms. Alcohol withdrawal can also cause seizures. Alcohol withdrawal is a serious medical condition that can be fatal. Hospitalization and treatment with benzodiazepines such as diazepam (Valium®) or chlordiazepoxide (Librium®) are usually necessary for alcohol withdrawal and may be lifesaving.

Who Gets Alcoholic Liver Disease?

Most individuals with liver disease caused by alcohol probably suffer from alcohol dependence. However, some individuals who have abused alcohol over many years may also develop liver disease. It is also possible that individuals who do not strictly meet the diagnostic criteria for either of these conditions will develop liver disease after many years of drinking. There are multiple genetic and environmental factors that determine if a person who consumes alcohol is at risk for liver disease, most of which have not been identified.

An alcoholic "drink" generally contains 10 g of alcohol. This is roughly the amount of alcohol in a 12 oz. bottle of beer, a glass (4 oz.) of wine, or 1.5 oz. of distilled spirits. There is no magic number of drinks a day that cause alcoholic liver disease. Probably two alcoholic drinks a day for many years is the conservative minimum amount necessary to develop alcohol-related liver disease. Six or more alcoholic drinks every day significantly increases the risk for developing liver disease. Some individuals, however, will never develop liver disease no matter how much alcohol they consume. For reasons that remain unclear, women appear to be more likely to develop liver disease than men at relatively low amounts of daily alcohol consumption. It should also be realized that alcohol consumption can cause serious social and physical problems other than liver disease. Therefore, the risk for developing liver disease from alcohol is not the only reason to limit alcohol consumption. Perhaps the most important aspect of alcoholic liver disease is that once a patient develops liver disease from alcohol consumption, that individual is drinking too much and should never drink again.

The Spectrum of Alcoholic Liver Disease

Excessive alcohol consumption causes three different liver disorders: fatty liver, alcoholic hepatitis, and cirrhosis. Fatty liver and alcoholic hepatitis are completely reversible if the patient stops drinking. Cirrhosis (see chapter 3) is not reversible, yet cessation of alcohol consumption can prevent liver function in a patient with alcoholic cirrhosis from deteriorating further. Any combination of fatty liver, alcoholic hepatitis, and cirrhosis can occur simultaneously in the liver of someone who consumes excessive alcohol. A common example is the occurrence of alcoholic hepatitis in an individual who starts a binge of heavier drinking and already has cirrhosis caused by alcohol. Although cirrhosis is not reversible, this individual's condition may improve dramatically upon cessation of alcohol consumption as the hepatitis resolves itself.

Fatty liver

Excessive alcohol consumption can lead to the accumulation of fat in liver cells. The individual with fatty liver caused by alcohol usually does not have physical signs or symptoms of liver disease. He or she may suffer from nonspecific symptoms such as fatigue. Fatty liver can cause blood test abnormalities and usually mild elevations in the blood AST and/or ALT activities. A diagnosis of fatty liver can be made with certainty only by liver biopsy. Fatty liver caused by alcohol will resolve itself if the patient stops drinking. In the examples given at the start of this section, the patient described in case 3 likely had fatty liver from alcohol that later resolved itself.

Alcoholic hepatitis

Excessive alcohol consumption can cause hepatitis or inflammation of the liver. Clinically, alcoholic hepatitis can range from relatively mild illness with fever, pain in the right upper abdomen, nausea, and vomiting to a severe life-threatening condition. Blood AST and ALT activities are usually elevated. In alcohol hepatitis, AST activity is frequently two or more times higher than ALT activity. In severe cases, alcoholic hepatitis can cause many of the same complications as cirrhosis including ascites, hepatic encephalopathy, and bleeding esophageal varices. If these complications are caused by alcoholic hepatitis, they will reverse themselves as the inflammation resolves if the individual stops drinking. In contrast, they will not reverse if caused by cirrhosis. The patient described in case 1 is an example of someone with both cirrhosis and alcoholic hepatitis.

When examined under the microscope, liver inflammation caused by alcohol appears very different than liver inflammation caused by hepatitis viruses or most other drugs. The inflammation of alcoholic hepatitis can be readily distinguished from these other types by performing a liver biopsy. However, liver biopsy is usually not necessary in patients with alcoholic hepatitis as the diagnosis is readily made based upon typical symptoms in a patient with excessive alcohol consumption. Once the clinical symptoms of alcoholic hepatitis resolve themselves, liver biopsy may be indicated to determine the presence underlying cirrhosis.

Cirrhosis

Chronic consumption of excessive amounts of alcohol can cause cirrhosis (see chapter 3). In the U.S., alcohol is the number one cause of cirrhosis. Very often, cirrhosis will be the initial presentation of a patient with alcohol liver disease. This is exemplified by the hypothetical patient in case 2.

Effects of Alcohol on Metabolism by the Liver

Excessive alcohol consumption affects its own metabolism plus that of other drugs by the liver. In most individuals, alcohol is primarily broken down by enzymes known as alcohol dehydrogenases. These enzymes speed up the chemical reaction that converts ethyl alcohol to its metabolite acetaldehyde.

Acetaldehyde is an important metabolite of alcohol because it is associated with unpleasant effects such as flushing, nausea, and vomiting. It may also play a role in long-term liver damage caused by alcohol. In the body, acetaldehyde is metabolized to acetic acid (vinegar) by a chemical reaction enhanced by the enzyme known as aldehyde dehydrogenase. An individual with a genetic deficiency of aldehyde dehydrogenase, which is not uncommon in persons of Asian descent, becomes red and warm after just a few sips of alcohol. Pharmacological inhibition of aldehyde dehydrogenase is also accomplished by the drug disulfram (Antabuse®). This drug is sometimes taken by individuals with alcohol use disorders to deter them from drinking as they will feel sick after consuming alcohol due to acetaldehyde buildup.

Chronic excessive alcohol consumption induces synthesis of an enzyme in the liver known as cytochrome P450 (actually a family of related enzymes). Cytochrome P450 can metabolize alcohol and it becomes a major pathway for alcohol metabolism in the chronic alcohol drinker. Oxidation of alcohol by cytochrome P450 utilizes certain cofactors in the cell at a high rate. This influences the body's overall metabolism and may play some role in causing liver and other organ dysfunction. Induction of cytochrome P450 also explains, in part, the "tolerance" to alcohol present in some individuals with alcohol dependence. Because alcohol is more readily metabolized in the liver by cytochrome P450, it takes more alcohol to achieve a desired blood concentration.

Cytochrome P450 enzymes metabolize other drugs besides alcohol. For this reason, the doses of some drugs must be adjusted in alcoholics. Some drugs become relatively ineffective in the alcoholic as cytochrome P450 catalyzes their breakdown into harmless metabolites that are excreted. Other drugs may potentially become more toxic in heavy alcohol drinkers if the metabolites that result from the action of cytochrome P450 are toxic. There are hundreds of drugs whose metabolism is influenced by alcohol.

Effects of Alcohol on Other Parts of the Body

Alcohol affects many organs of the body besides the liver, and disorders can occur in individuals without liver disease. Frequently, individuals with alcoholic liver disease also have problems with other organ systems resulting from excessive alcohol consumption. These problems can complicate the clinical picture of the individual with alcoholic liver disease. The complicating problems frequently observed in individuals with alcoholic liver disease include:

Nervous system

Alcohol obviously affects the brain and its intoxicating effects due to excessive consumption are familiar to virtually everyone. Individuals with alcohol dependence may develop a tolerance to alcohol's intoxicating effects. Some component of tolerance is metabolic in that alcohol is more readily metabolized by induced cytochrome P450 enzymes. However, some component of tolerance to alcohol's intoxicating effects occur because of nerve cell structure changes. The resulting higher concentrations of blood become necessary to alter brain function. A component of tolerance to alcohol is also behavioral as chronic alcohol drinkers "learn" how to perform certain tasks while intoxicated.

Chronic alcohol consumption also affects the brain in more severe ways. Many alcohol-dependent individuals eventually become deficient in thiamine (vitamin B1). Thiamine deficiency can lead to a serious neuropsychiatric condition known as Wernicke-Korsakoff syndrome. Structural changes are observed in particular parts of the brain in individuals with this condition, and the syndrome has two separate components that often occur together but can be seen separately: Wernicke encephalopathy and Korsakoff psychosis. Wernicke encephalopathy is characterized by profound alterations in brain function. It can be diagnosed on physical examination by abnormal function of one of the nerves that moves the eye in certain directions. Korsakoff psychosis is a dramatic psychiatric condition characterized by confabulation (making up stories) and loss of some memory functions, usually of more recent events. Wernicke-

Korsakoff syndrome can complicate the overall clinical picture of a patient with alcoholic liver disease. It can also combine with hepatic encephalopathy and alcohol withdrawal symptoms resulting in complex neurological problems. Treatment with thiamine usually reverses Wernicke encephalopathy but does not always improve the memory disturbances associated with Korsakoff psychosis.

Alcohol has other effects on the nervous system. It can damage peripheral nerves and cause loss of sensation. Chronic alcohol consumption can cause cerebellar degeneration or loss of nerve cells in the cerebellum, the portion of the brain that regulates coordination. Finally, years of excessive alcohol consumption can cause diffuse loss of nerve cells in the brain and generalized dementia.

Gastrointestinal system

Alcohol can cause disease in other parts of the gastrointestinal system besides the liver. Alcohol causes pancreatitis, or inflammation of the pancreas. This is characterized by severe abdominal or back pain, fever, and inability to eat or digest certain foods. Pancreatitis can be life threatening and require hospitalization and even intensive care. Alcohol also causes gastritis and possibly stomach and duodenal ulcers. Gastritis and ulcers can complicate the diagnosis of gastrointestinal bleeding in an individual with alcoholic liver disease because the chances of bleeding from esophageal varices, gastritis, or stomach ulcers are all increased in the alcoholic. Emergency endoscopic examination of an alcoholic is almost always required to diagnose sources of bleeding in the stomach, esophagus, or intestines. Alcohol can also cause excessive vomiting and retching. The result can be tears in the esophagus that can bleed (Mallory-Weiss tears).

Heart and muscle

Excessive alcohol consumption can affect the heart and muscles. *Cardiomyopathy*, characterized by decreased effectiveness of heart pumping and an enlarged heart, is possible. Abnormal heart rhythms can also result from alcohol consumption and withdrawal. Further, alcohol can cause a myopathy or inflammation of the skeletal muscles leading to weakness.

Blood

Alcohol suppresses the bone marrow where blood cells are made. Chronic alcohol drinkers may become anemic from alcohol consumption and also have low white blood counts. Alcohol can directly lower the platelet count and further decrease it in cirrhotic individuals who may also have low platelet counts secondary to trapping of platelets in an enlarged spleen. Low platelets can cause a tendency to bleed.

Other complications

Excessive alcohol drinkers are also at risk for other complications. They include:

- *Falls and injuries*—An old radiologist's tale says that "the radiological diagnosis of alcoholism is made by finding multiple broken ribs on a chest X-ray." Head injuries from falls can result in skull fractures and cause bleeding in the space around the brain (subdural hematoma).
- *Infections*—Because alcoholics are often in a stupor or near-unconscious state, they are at risk for aspirating vomit into their lungs that can cause serious pneumonia (aspiration pneumonia). Because their immune systems may be compromised, alcoholics are also at increased risk for infections from bacteria that do not usually infect healthy individuals.

- *Predisposition to certain cancers*—Long-term heavy alcohol use increases the chances of developing throat cancer. Because the large majority of individuals who abuse alcohol also abuse tobacco, many are also at increased risk for development of lung cancer. The combination of tobacco and alcohol together make the risk for developing throat cancer even higher.
- *Psychosocial problems*—Individuals with alcohol use disorders have higher rates of psychosocial problems such as unemployment, poverty, homelessness, and incarceration for crimes.

Individuals with alcohol use disorders are at risk for many problems in addition to liver disease. Because of alcohol's multiple negative effects on the body, the management of individuals with alcoholic liver disease presents one of medicine's greatest challenges. This challenge is complicated even further by the alcoholic's inevitable psychological and social problems.

Diagnosis of Alcoholic Liver Disease

A history of excessive alcohol consumption in a patient with liver abnormalities suggests a diagnosis of alcoholic liver disease. The diagnosis can sometimes be made clinically when a patient with a known alcohol dependence disorder presents with signs, symptoms, and laboratory abnormalities of liver disease. However, other causes of liver disease, such as chronic viral hepatitis, drugs, and congenital disorders should not be excluded as patients who consume excessive amounts of alcohol may also have these problems. Sometimes, a history of alcohol consumption is difficult to obtain from a patient or family members, and individuals with alcohol use disorders *are notorious for lying about the amount of alcohol they consume.* A general rule is that the patient usually consumes at least three times more alcohol than he or she tells the doctor. In these cases, various laboratory tests may suggest excessive alcohol consumption. The blood GGTP activity may be elevated from alcohol consumption and the mean corpuscular volume of red blood cells may be decreased. In patients with alcoholic hepatitis, blood AST activity may be two or more times higher than blood ALT activity whereas in other forms of hepatitis ALT and AST activities are roughly equal.

If a diagnosis of alcoholic liver disease cannot be made on clinical grounds, liver biopsy may be necessary. For example, in the patient with a questionable history of alcohol abuse who presents to the doctor with elevated blood AST and ALT activities, liver biopsy may be necessary to diagnose fatty liver, alcoholic hepatitis, or cirrhosis. Liver biopsy may also be necessary to establish the presence of cirrhosis if it is not clinically apparent. Old studies have shown that liver biopsy reveals a liver disease other than alcohol liver disease in about 25 percent of patients who drink and in whom alcoholic liver disease is suspected by clinical criteria. Therefore, liver biopsy is also helpful to exclude another or concurrent liver disorder in a person with an alcohol abuse disorder.

Treatment

The cornerstone of treatment of an individual with alcoholic liver disease is *complete and unconditional abstinence from alcohol.* This cannot be emphasized enough. Fatty liver and alcoholic hepatitis will resolve themselves if alcohol consumption is stopped. Cirrhosis is not reversible; however, the patient's condition may improve and not progress if he or she stops drinking alcohol.

Abstinence from alcohol is often easier said than done. Substance abuse and dependence are diseases, and a component of these diseases is an inability to stop using the substance despite knowing it is harmful. Individuals with alcohol dependence may suffer withdrawal upon stopping drinking and this can prove fatal. Hospital admission for detoxification may therefore be required for alcohol-dependent individuals. In many cases, detoxification should ideally be followed up by inpatient rehabilitation for at least one month. Additional outpatient psychotherapy is often necessary and participation in Alcoholics Anonymous should probably be continued for life. Despite this course of action, the relapse rate is quite high.

Supportive medical care may be necessary for the patient with alcoholic liver disease. Complications of cirrhosis are treated as described in chapter 3. Acute alcohol hepatitis may require hospitalization and treatment. Some studies suggest that steroids may be beneficial in severe cases, and other complications caused by alcohol such as gastritis may also respond to treatment. Although medical treatment is often essential to support patients with alcohol-related illnesses, *no medication or procedure is a substitute for abstinence in the treatment of alcoholic liver disease.*

Drugs and Toxins

Many drugs can cause liver disease. The signs and symptoms associated with liver damage induced by drugs or toxins can vary tremendously. Many patients will have no obvious problems and liver damage can only be ascertained by blood testing. Some patients will have no symptoms for years and eventually develop cirrhosis from chronic drug use or toxin exposure. Some drug-induced liver diseases will present as fulminant hepatic failure.

It is extremely important that doctors and patients realize that many different drugs can cause liver damage. A comprehensive history regarding medications—both prescription and over-the-counter—is an essential part of evaluating a patient with liver disease. In older adults, prescription medications are a major cause of liver abnormalities picked up on routine blood tests suggesting liver diseases (elevated blood aminotransferase, alkaline phosphatase, and GGTP activities). One intelligent approach when faced with a patient on medications causing liver problems is to realize that a drug may be causing liver disease or blood test abnormality. This can sometimes be established by the known adverse event profile of a drug plus excluding other disorders. Another way to determine if a drug is causing a liver problem is for the doctor (*not* the patient without the doctor's knowledge) to discontinue it. If the abnormality resolves itself, the drug is likely the culprit. Restarting the drug and witnessing return of the abnormality strongly suggests this.

After a drug is established to be the cause of liver disease, the decision to stop or continue use of the drug requires the judgment of an experienced physician. For example, mild cholestasis indicated by slightly elevated blood alkaline phosphatase and GGTP activities may be less significant than the repercussions of stopping a medication to prevent seizures or psychosis. On the other hand, continued use of a particular agent to lower blood pressure that is causing hepatitis may not be reasonable if equally effective alternative drugs are available. Therefore, the doctor's experience and judgment are critical in deciding if the risk of continuing a drug affecting the liver outweighs the potential danger. It is not possible to provide specific guidelines for these decisions.

Overdoses of certain drugs or exposure to certain toxins can also cause acute liver disease and even fulminant hepatic failure. Some individuals may also have unusual (idiosyncratic) reactions that can cause severe liver disease with normal doses of a generally safe drug, an example being the anesthetic halothane. In these cases, the goal is to identify the cause of the liver disease, immediately stop the drug or toxin if exposure is ongoing, and support the patient until liver function recovers.

It is difficult to provide an exhaustive list of drugs and compounds that affect the liver because there are thousands that affect it in many different ways. In this section, I will discuss only liver toxicities associated with commonly used drugs and classical hepatotoxins (see Table 4.1).

Acetaminophen

Acetaminophen is the active ingredient in many over-the-counter pain relievers including Tylenol®. At recommended doses and durations of treatment, acetaminophen is an extremely safe compound used by millions of people worldwide. Despite a few unconfirmed case reports in the literature, there are no controlled studies showing that acetaminophen is toxic to the liver when taken as recommended on package labels. An overdose of acetaminophen, however, is another matter.

Overdose of acetaminophen, which is also known as paracetamol in some parts of the world, was first recognized as a method for committing suicide in Great Britain and later in the U.S. Overdoses of acetaminophen, usually more than 15 g at a time in adults (each "extra-strength" tablet or capsule contains half a gram), can cause fulminant hepatic failure. Some individuals have been reported to have taken overdoses of acetamino-

Table 4.1. *Some commonly used drugs that can affect the liver and examples of classical hepatotoxins.*

Drugs	Acetaminophen overdose
	Isoniazid (INH)
	"Statins"
	Halothane
	Methotrexate
	Anticonvulsants
	Phenytoin (Dilantin®)
	Valproic acid
	Psychiatric medications
	Cancer chemotherapy
	Antihypertensive agents
	Alpha-methyldopa
	Cardiovascular drugs
	Antidiabetic agents
	Estrogens (birth control pills)
	Anabolic steroids
Classical hepatotoxic compounds	*Amanita phalloides* mushrooms (death caps)
	Carbon tetrachloride
	Pyrrolizidine alkaloids
	Jamaican bush tea

phen with "therapeutic intent" and not as deliberate suicide attempts. Therefore, in patients with acute liver disease of unclear etiology, a very careful history of all over-the-counter drug use (acetaminophen is in many over-the-counter products) and amounts consumed is extremely important.

The diagnosis of acetaminophen overdose is usually made by history and detection of toxic levels in the blood. The time of ingestion must be known to determine if the blood level is toxic. The clinical picture of acetaminophen overdose can be one of massive liver cell death. This will be manifested by extremely high blood aminotransferase activities within a couple of days after the overdose that rapidly return to normal. Signs and symptoms of liver failure usually first occur about two days later. Some patients, however, will not develop serious liver damage, even with large doses.

N-acetylcysteine (Mucomyst®) is the treatment for acetaminophen overdose. It has been hypothesized that N-acetylcysteine's mechanism of action is to neutralize a toxic metabolite of acetaminophen that at normal concentrations is easily detoxified by the liver. N-acetylcysteine is most effective if given within ten hours of an acetaminophen overdose and probably not effective if given more than twenty-four hours later. For patients who develop fulminant hepatic failure from acetaminophen overdose, intensive care is essential and emergent liver transplantation may be necessary.

Isoniazid

Isoniazid, or INH, is widely used in the treatment and prevention of tuberculosis. People with active tuberculosis, and many with only positive skin tests, are treated with isoniazid. Treatment usually lasts for six months. About 10 percent of individuals treated with isoniazid develop transient, mild elevations in blood aminotransferase activities. These are not serious and treatment can be continued. However, about 1 percent of individuals develop severe hepatitis and some even develop fulminant hepatic failure.

Isoniazid hepatitis is rare in younger individuals but occurs in about 2 percent of treated individuals over age fifty. In active tuberculosis, the risk of no treatment is far greater than the risk of liver disease from isoniazid. A more conservative approach may be used in individuals with positive skin tests in whom isoniazid is prescribed to prevent active tuberculosis, however. The decision depends upon the individual's risk factors for developing active tuberculosis and must be made by the patient's doctor using guidelines recommended by public health agencies or professional organizations.

"Statins"

The HMG-CoA reductase inhibitor "statin" class of drugs are used to lower serum cholesterol concentrations. These are some of the most widely prescribed drugs in the U.S. This class of compounds includes lovastatin (Mevacor®), pravastatin (Pravachol®), simvastatin (Zocor®), fluvastatin (Lescol®), atorvastatin (Lipitor®), and cerivastatin (Baychol®). Hepatitis, as presumed from increases in blood aminotransferase activities, occurs in about 1 percent of patients receiving starting doses of these drugs and in up to 2 percent of those who receive maximum doses. Patients are usually asymptomatic. Those who receive statins should have their aminotransferase activities checked by blood testing four to six weeks after first taking the drug or increasing dosage. They should also be checked periodically while on the medications. If blood ALT or AST activities persistently increase to more than three times normal, the medications should probably be discontinued. Any liver inflammation induced by statins is reversible upon stopping the drugs.

Halothane

Halothane has been widely used over the years as a general anesthetic. In about 1 in 10,000 cases, halothane causes hepatitis. The onset of hepatitis usually begins a few days to within three weeks after receiving anesthesia. Halothane can induce a mild hepatitis that is detectable only by finding elevated blood aminotransferase activities, or fatal fulminant hepatic failure. Almost all patients with halothane-induced hepatitis have had prior exposure to the drug, and repeated exposure greatly increases the chance of developing hepatitis. Therefore, halothane should be avoided in individuals for whom repeated surgeries are anticipated or who have been exposed previously to the drug. The anesthetics methoxyflurane and enflurane may also cause hepatitis similar to that caused by halothane.

Methotrexate

Methotrexate is commonly used to treat severe psoriasis and other rheumatic diseases. Chronic therapy with methotrexate can cause fibrosis (scarring) and cirrhosis of the liver. These changes are dose-related and most studies show that cirrhosis is rare with total cumulative doses of less than 1.5 g. Methotrexate can cause liver damage without causing abnormalities in the aminotransferase activities or other blood tests. For this reason, liver biopsy to determine fibrosis is sometimes performed after a cumulative dose of 1 to 1.5 g of methotrexate.

Anticonvulsants

Two commonly used anticonvulsants (drugs to prevent seizures) can cause liver disease. Phenytoin (Dilantin) causes various types of liver damage. Its continued use, if liver abnormalities occur, depends upon the risk of recurrent seizures and availability of alternative effective drugs compared to continued treatment. Rare cases of acute phenytoin liver injury have been reported that can cause fulminant hepatic failure. Valproic acid (Depekote®) and its derivatives can also cause liver disease. Mild elevations in blood aminotransferase activities are not uncommon and should be followed by repeated blood testing. Valproic acid can also cause clinically significant liver disease. Valproic acid liver damage is characterized by death of liver cells and accumulation of microscopic fat globules in liver cells.

Psychiatric Medications

Various drugs used in the treatment of psychiatric disorders can affect the liver. Phenothiazines such as chlorpromazine (Thorazine®) that are used to treat schizophrenia and other forms of psychosis commonly cause cholestasis or impaired bile flow within the liver. This can lead to jaundice. Elevations in the blood alkaline phosphatase and GGTP activities are often the first indications of this disorder. Some antidepressant medications can cause hepatitis, and are usually inferred from elevations in blood ALT and AST activities. Continued use of drugs for these conditions depends upon the risk of their discontinuation causing life-threatening mood changes or psychotic behavior versus the slight risk of progressive liver damage. Sometimes one type of drug can be substituted for another. This decision will doubtless depend upon careful collaboration between the psychiatrist and liver specialist.

Cancer Chemotherapy

Many drugs used for cancer chemotherapy can cause different types of liver damage. An interesting condition caused by high dose chemotherapy with several different agents is known as *veno-occlusive disease*. Veno-occlusive disease is characterized by damage that causes obstruction of the smallest hepatic veins that exit the liver. Acute veno-occlusive disease can mimic hepatic vein obstruction and clinically present as the sudden onset of abdominal discomfort, enlarged liver, and ascites. Slowly progressive courses can also occur. There is no specific treatment.

Antihypertensive Agents

Several drugs used to control blood pressure can cause liver damage. A classic example is alpha-methyldopa (Aldomet®), though this drug is rarely used today. Rare cases of liver damage have been associated with a variety of other blood pressure medications.

Cardiovascular Drugs

Various drugs used to treat heart disease have also been associated with liver toxicity. Many heart drugs can potentially cause hepatitis, but occurrence is rare considering how frequently such drugs are prescribed. One culprit that causes a unique form of liver disease is amiodarone, which is used to treat heart rhythm abnormalities. Amiodarone liver toxicity is problematic because it is sometimes associated with no clinical or laboratory evidence of liver disease until significant damage has occurred. Upon liver biopsy, unusual fatty inclusions are often observed.

Antidiabetic Agents

Various oral medications used to treat diabetes mellitus can cause liver damage. Troglitazone (Rezulin®), a relatively new and very effective drug used by diabetics, has been reported to cause serious liver disease and even fulminant hepatic failure. Fortunately, cases of severe liver disease have been rare considering troglitazone's widespread use. Blood aminotransferase activities should be checked at the start of therapy, monthly for the first eight months of therapy, every two months for the remainder of the first year, and periodically thereafter. The drug should be discontinued if clinical evidence of liver disease develops or if blood ALT activity increases to more than one-and-a-half times normal.

Birth Control Pills and Other Estrogen Preparations

Estrogens, most commonly present in birth control pills and medications used to treat symptoms of menopause, can cause cholestasis (impaired bile flow in the small bile ducts in the liver). This is characterized by itching over the body, possibly jaundice, and elevations in blood alkaline phosphatase and

GGTP activities. Cholestasis typically occurs within the first two months of taking birth control pills. Birth control pill use has also been associated with various liver tumors, including benign adenomas and another benign condition known as focal nodular hyperplasia. These conditions are rare.

Anabolic Steroids and Androgens

Anabolic steroids are sometimes used by body builders and athletes to enhance results. Anabolic steroid use has been associated with a condition known as peliosis hepatitis, which are blood-filled spaces in the liver devoid of cells. Increased incidence of a rare form of liver cancer due to anabolic steroid use may also occur.

Hepatotoxins

Various toxins can cause liver disease. Toxins that damage the liver are referred to as *hepatotoxins* or *hepatotoxic* substances. The most dramatic hepatotoxins are those that cause severe acute disease or fulminant hepatic failure. A classic example is *Amanita phalloides* mushrooms, also known as death caps, which can cause fulminant hepatic failure. Another classic example is ingestion of carbon tetrachloride, which used to be present in cleaning fluids and can cause sudden hepatic necrosis and fulminant hepatic failure.

Pyrrolizidine causes liver veno-occlusive disease similar to that caused by various cancer chemotherapeutic agents. Pyrrolizidine toxicity is perhaps most commonly caused by traditional medicines or bush teas prepared in the West Indies. Pyrrolizidine poisoning is not uncommon in Jamaica, where medicinal bush teas prepared from poisonous plants are sometimes given to children.

Although virtually nonexistent in the U.S., aflatoxins are a common cause of chronic liver disease in other parts of the world, especially tropical regions. Aflatoxins are produced by a mold that is a contaminant of a variety of nuts (most commonly peanuts), beans, and grains. Chronic aflatoxin ingestion can cause cirrhosis. Of most concern throughout the world is the role that chronic ingestion of aflatoxins and their metabolites have in the development of hepatocellular carcinoma (primary liver cancer).

The A, B, C's (D, E, and G?) of Viral Hepatitis

Hepatitis means inflammation of the liver. By now, it should be obvious that there are many causes of hepatitis, including drugs and alcohol. However, most people equate the term *hepatitis* with the liver disease caused by several different viruses. Hepatitis caused by a virus is more precisely called *viral hepatitis.*

After alcohol, viral hepatitis is the leading cause of chronic liver disease in the U.S. It is estimated that, at the present time, about one million Americans are chronically infected with hepatitis B virus and four million with hepatitis C virus. Worldwide, viral hepatitis surpasses alcohol as the number one cause of chronic liver disease. About 300 million people, mostly in Southeast Asia and sub-Saharan Africa, are chronically infected with hepatitis B virus. Perhaps as many as 150 million individuals worldwide are chronically infected with hepatitis C virus. These numbers are staggering, especially since hepatitis B and hepatitis C are infectious diseases whose transmission can be prevented by avoiding certain behaviors and using some commonsense precautions. Hepatitis B can also be prevented by vaccination.

Because of advances in basic molecular biology, and the large numbers of affected individuals, diagnosis and treatment of viral hepatitis is currently the most active area of medicine related to diseases of the liver. The different forms of viral hepatitis are also the liver diseases about which most patients seem to have questions. Our knowledge of viral hepatitis is still expanding, especially regarding hepatitis C, which was identified only about ten years ago. However, currently available information makes it possible to understand a good deal about the major hepatitis viruses and the diseases that each causes.

What Is a Virus?

Before discussing the various types of viral hepatitis, it is important to have some understanding of what a virus is. This will hopefully provide some idea as to why viral diseases are formidable problems. So sit tight and try to bear with a little basic biochemistry and cell biology.

Some people define viruses as the simplest forms of life. It is really a matter of philosophical debate—and not science—to decide if viruses are "alive." Like other life forms, viruses reproduce and mutate (randomly change their genetic material). However, *viruses do not have an independent metabolism and can replicate only within cells.* You can decide for yourself if this constitutes life.

Virus are small and range in size from about 15 nanometers to 250 nanometers in their longest dimension. There are a billion nanometers in a meter, which is roughly equal to one yard. The human red blood cell, one of the smallest cells in the body, is about thirty times the size of the largest virus. Hepatocytes, the predominant liver cells, are much larger than the various hepatitis viruses. Particles as small as viruses cannot be observed under a light microscope. Electron microscopy is necessary to see virus particles.

Viruses contain either ribonucleic acid (RNA) or deoxyribonucleic acid (DNA) as their genetic material (animals and plants have DNA as their genetic material). Viruses also contain proteins. Most viruses have core or capsid proteins that form a nucleocapsid around which the viral RNA or DNA winds. Some viruses are enveloped in that they contain a lipid (fatty) outer layer that derives from the cells in which they replicate. The envelope usually contains specific viral proteins. For examples of how some viruses look, see the diagrams of the hepatitis B virus (Figure 4.1) and hepatitis C virus (Figure 4.5) later in this chapter. In addition to the proteins that comprise the viral particle, most viruses also produce proteins that perform essential biochemical functions necessary for their replication. These "nonstructural" proteins may be expressed and function only within the cells that the virus infects and not present in the mature viral particles.

An important property of viruses is cellular *tropism*. Tropism indicates a virus's ability to infect a particular type of cell or cells. Viruses that cause hepatitis are referred to as *primarily hepatotropic* because they preferentially infect hepatocytes, the major cells of the liver. Primarily hepatotropic viruses may also infect other cells beside hepatocytes. Various viruses have different cellular tropisms. For example, the human immunodeficiency virus (HIV) primarily infects certain cells of the immune system.

Another important property of viruses is their ability to mutate. Because the genomes of viruses are small and replicate rapidly, the mutation rates of viruses are usually high. The ability of viruses to mutate is of critical importance in their ability to cause disease. Constant mutation allows viruses to escape detection by the host's immune system. For this reason, it is sometimes not possible for the body to clear a viral infection. Mutation may be an important way that hepatitis C virus escapes detection by the immune system. Mutation also makes it difficult to design drugs against viruses as they can cause changes in the viral proteins that are targets for drugs.

Latency is another property of viruses that is of major significance for treatment of human diseases. Viruses may stop replicating and integrate their DNA, or a DNA copy of their RNA, into the host cell DNA. In this manner, the virus can be propagated as the host cell divides. However, viral particles will not be made and the immune system will usually not kill the cells in which viral genetic material is integrated. A latent or integrated virus can later be activated for various reasons and begin to replicate and make infectious viral particles. This is an important property of the hepatitis B virus that can either replicate in infected individuals at high levels or integrate into the cell's DNA and replicate at a very low level.

Viruses do not have their own independent metabolism and utilize the energy, chemical compounds, and protein synthesis machinery of the cells they infect. For this reason, it has been an extremely difficult task to design antiviral drugs. Antibiotics that kill bacteria are often targeted against the bacterial proteins involved in protein synthesis or energy metabolism. Since viruses use host cell metabolites and protein synthesis machinery, drugs directed against these targets would not only inhibit viral replication but also kill host cells. Fortunately, some viruses make a few proteins that are uniquely essential for their own replication that can be targets for antiviral drugs. An example that has received a lot of attention in recent years is the protease of HIV, which is a viral protein essential for replication of the virus that is the target of drugs known as protease inhibitors.

In sum, viruses can be considered as tiny cellular parasites (whether they are alive or not is not really an issue). Viruses infect cells and utilize their energy sources, chemical compounds, and protein synthesis machinery to replicate themselves. Many viruses can live quietly inside cells for many years without replicating and can be activated at any time. They use various tricks, including rapid mutation, to evade the host's immune system so that they can live in the host for a long time (ideally for the virus, a lifetime). The relationship between most viruses and hosts is not mutual, however, and virus infection in humans often leads to disease and sometimes death. This is because either the virus itself, or the immune response directed against infected cells, kills all cells infected with a virus.

The Major Human Hepatotropic Viruses

There are five major human hepatotropic viruses: hepatitis A virus, hepatitis B virus, hepatitis C virus, hepatitis D virus, and hepatitis E virus (Table 4.2). The diseases they cause are known as hepatitis A, hepatitis B, hepatitis C, hepatitis D, and hepatitis E, respectively. Papers published in 1995 and 1996 reported discovery of a virus known as hepatitis G virus that is commonly present in the blood supply and has been detected in individuals with acute and chronic hepatitis. Today, most investigators feel that hepatitis G virus does not cause acute or chronic hepatitis. This is not entirely clear, however. It certainly does not appear to be a major cause of liver disease. There is no "hepatitis F" virus.

The different human hepatitis viruses are actually *very* different. They also cause different types of liver disease, and there are several possible ways to classify them. Virologists may classify them based on the sequences of their DNA and RNA or

Table 4.2. The major human hepatitis viruses.

Virus	Genetic Material	Family	Disease	Major Modes of Transmission
Hepatitis A	RNA	*Picornaviridae*	Acute hepatitis	Contaminated food and water
Hepatitis B	DNA	*Hepadnaviridae*	Acute and chronic hepatitis	Blood; mother to infant; sex
Hepatitis C	RNA	*Flaviviridae*	Acute and chronic hepatitis	Blood; mother to infant; and sex less efficiently
Hepatitis D	RNA	*Deltaviridae*	Acute and chronic hepatitis	Blood (only infection along with hepatitis B)
Hepatitis E	RNA	*Caliciviridae*	Acute hepatitis	Contaminated food and water

based upon the families of related viruses to which they belong. Clinicians may prefer to classify them by the types of hepatitis they cause. Epidemiologists may be more interested in the ways they are transmitted. Table 4.2 lists some of the characteristics of the five major human hepatitis viruses.

Hepatitis A

Definition and symptoms

The illness caused by infection from the hepatitis A virus is called hepatitis A. In the past, several different terms were used to describe this illness. These included infectious hepatitis, epidemic hepatitis, epidemic jaundice, catarrhal jaundice, and infectious icterus. These terms are generally no longer used.

The hepatitis A virus causes only acute liver disease. This is critical to understand as many patients, and even some doctors, consider hepatitis A a possible cause of chronic liver disease. Individuals with other chronic liver diseases, as might any susceptible individual, can be infected with hepatitis A virus and develop acute hepatitis. However, hepatitis A virus does not cause chronic liver disease. Hepatitis A always resolves itself or, in rare cases, kills the patient.

In most patients, hepatitis A is either a relatively mild disease or no apparent disease at all. Many children who get infected do not develop clinically apparent liver disease. There is a correlation between age and disease severity. Most cases of fulminant hepatic failure from hepatitis A virus infection occurs in older individuals, usually over age fifty. Patients with a relatively mild form of the disease may suffer from nausea, vomiting, fever, fatigue, and loss of appetite. Blood tests usually reveal elevations in aminotransferase activities and possible elevations in bilirubin concentration. Patients with a more severe hepatitis A condition develop jaundice and laboratory examination reveals significant elevation in blood bilirubin concentration. In more severe cases, prothrombin time may be prolonged. In instances of massive hepatocyte death, blood ALT and AST activities can be very highly elevated.

The large majority of patients with hepatitis A recover without complications. Hospitalization and supportive care may be necessary for very ill patients who are unable to eat or drink fluids. Occasionally, patients may suffer from fatigue and malaise for several months after the disease resolves. About 1 percent of individuals with hepatitis A, usually those over age fifty, develop serious liver failure, sometimes fulminant. These patients require hospitalization and supportive care. In the U.S., about 1 in 300 cases of hepatitis A results in death or emergency liver transplantation.

Transmission

Hepatitis A virus is spread primarily by the fecal-oral route. The virus is excreted in feces of infected people and infects susceptible individuals who consume contaminated water or foods. Water, shellfish, and salads are the most frequently implicated sources of transmission. Cold cuts, fruits, fruit juices, milk, and vegetables have also been implicated in various outbreaks. Hepatitis A is more common in underdeveloped parts of the world with poor sanitary conditions. Travelers to these regions are at an increased risk for infection.

The time from infection with hepatitis A virus to onset of symptoms varies from ten to fifty days. Thirty days is the average. The greatest danger of infecting others occurs during the middle of the incubation period and before presentation of symptoms. The patient remains potentially infectious up until a week or more after the onset of symptoms.

Although ingestion of contaminated food and water is the most common route of transmission, hepatitis A virus can be transmitted in other ways. Infected individuals can spread the virus to others who live in the same household or with whom they have sexual contact. In particular, hepatitis A virus may be spread by sexual practices in which the mouth comes in direct contact with the anal area of an infected individual. Homosexual men are at an increased risk for hepatitis A. Casual contact at work or in social settings usually does not spread the virus. Hepatitis A virus infection can, however, be spread among children and employees in child care centers where a child or employee is infected. Residents and staff workers in institutions for developmentally disabled persons are at a particularly increased risk for being infected with hepatitis A virus. There have also been reports of transmission by sharing contaminated materials among intravenous drug users.

In industrialized countries such as the U.S., hepatitis A often occurs in isolated outbreaks or epidemics. These outbreaks can usually be traced to contaminated foods. Foods implicated in hepatitis A outbreaks in the U.S. have included lettuce, raw oysters, other shellfish, and frozen strawberries.

Diagnosis

The diagnosis of hepatitis A is suspected when sudden onset of clinical liver disease is observed ten to fifty days after exposure to the hepatitis A virus. Diagnosis is confirmed by blood tests. The laboratory diagnosis of hepatitis A virus is made by detection of antibodies against the virus in the blood, and interpretation of blood test results is often tricky and requires some explanation. Patients who have been infected with hepatitis A develop two different types of antibodies against the virus. IgG antibodies are found in individuals who have been exposed at any time in the past. Hence the presence of IgG antibodies against hepatitis A is *not* diagnostic for acute infection and indicates past infection or exposure that may or may not have been accompanied by a recognized illness. Patients possessing IgG antibodies against the hepatitis A virus therefore become immune. IgM antibodies against hepatitis A virus are present only in acute hepatitis A, usually appearing within ten days of infection. The presence of IgM antibodies against the hepatitis A virus in someone with sudden onset liver disease is nearly 100 percent specific for the diagnosis of hepatitis A.

Treatment

There is no specific treatment for hepatitis A. In most cases, the disease is mild and self-limiting. As long as the patient is drinking and eating, hospitalization is generally not necessary. If the patient is so sick that he or she is vomiting extensively and cannot eat or drink, hospitalization may be necessary for administration of intravenous fluids. The patient can be discharged once he or she has adequate oral intake. In very serious cases, such as those causing fulminant hepatic failure, hospitalization and intensive care are required. Preferably, patients with fulminant hepatic failure should be hospitalized in medical centers where liver transplantation can be performed in case it becomes necessary.

Prevention

The most important issue regarding hepatitis A is prevention. There are three major ways to prevent hepatitis A. They are hygiene, passive immunity, and vaccination.

Hygienic measures to prevent hepatitis A infection concern preventing the contamination of food and water and avoiding contact with contaminated foods. In many developing countries, widespread sewage systems have not been constructed, especially in rural areas. Water from lakes and rivers into which people defecate may be used for drinking, washing, or preparing foods. Living conditions are often crowded. Only overall improvement in the socioeconomic structure can remedy these problems. Visitors to such areas should avoid drinking from the local water supply. They should also avoid eating fresh fruits or vegetables that may have been washed with water from local rivers, lakes, or reservoirs. Locally caught shellfish should not be consumed. If local water must be consumed, it should be boiled first.

People living in the same household as an individual with hepatitis A, or individuals working in situations where the disease is common, should follow commonsense rules. Hand washing should be strictly observed, especially when using the bathroom and before eating or preparing food. People working in child care centers or institutions for developmentally disabled individuals should wash their hands after changing diapers or sheets, before eating, or after any close contact with residents.

Passive immunization with immune globulin is recommended for short-term protection against hepatitis A and for persons who have been exposed to the hepatitis A virus. Immune globulin is a concentration of antibodies pooled from the blood of individuals with IgG antibodies against the hepatitis A virus. Immune globulin should be administered to individuals who will be traveling to endemic areas that have not received vaccination far enough in advance of departure (about four weeks) for it to be effective. The U.S. Centers for Disease Control and Prevention in Atlanta, Georgia (on the Internet, http://www.cdc.gov), provides recommendations for travelers going to various parts of the world. Immune globulin should also be given to individuals who may have been exposed to hepatitis A virus within two weeks of suspected exposure.

Hepatitis A vaccines provide long-term protection against hepatitis A. Two shots administered in six- to twelve-month intervals are given. Vaccination is recommended for individuals who will travel to or work in areas where hepatitis A is endemic. Again, the U.S. Centers for Disease Control and Prevention provides recommendations for travelers to various parts of the world. The first dose of vaccine should be given at least four weeks before travel. This usually provides protection for a short trip, but a booster is necessary six to twelve months later for long-term protection.

Children in communities with high rates of hepatitis A should also be vaccinated. These communities include Alaska Native villages, Native American reservations, and some religious communities, for example, the Kiryas Joel Hassidic community in New York. Homosexual men should also be vaccinated, as should persons who use street drugs. Individuals with chronic liver diseases should be vaccinated as hepatitis A virus infection may be more severe in individuals with another underlying liver disease. This may be particularly true for individuals with chronic hepatitis C. People with some other chronic diseases, such as inherited clotting factor deficiencies like hemophilia, should also be vaccinated. Hepatitis A vaccination is not recommended for all health care workers; however, those working in high-risk environments, such as institutions for the developmentally disabled, should receive the hepatitis A vaccine. Individuals who work with hepatitis A virus-infected animals, or with the hepatitis A virus in a research laboratory, should also be vaccinated.

People who have been previously infected with hepatitis A virus are generally immune to another infection and episode of hepatitis A. Immune individuals have serum IgG antibodies against the hepatitis A virus. Such people do not need to be vaccinated. However, it remains unclear whether it is more cost-effective to screen the blood of an at-risk individual for the presence of IgG antibodies or to just administer the vaccine.

Hepatitis B

Definition and symptoms

A little background on the virus that causes hepatitis B is essential for understanding the disease, its symptoms, and especially its diagnosis. The existence of hepatitis B virus was discovered by accident in the 1960s. In 1965, Dr. Baruch Blumberg and collaborators discovered a protein of the hepatitis B virus in the blood of an Australian aborigine. This protein was called the "Australia antigen." At the time of its discovery, the Australia antigen was not thought to be a viral protein. Over the next few years, however, Dr. Blumberg, his collaborators, and other groups proved that the Australia antigen was associated with hepatitis, specifically a form that was then known as "serum hepatitis" and was transmitted by blood. Dr. Blumberg was subsequently awarded the Nobel Prize in Medicine for this discovery.

In subsequent years, the hepatitis B virus was photographed under an electron microscope, propagated in cell culture, and its genetic material analyzed. A schematic diagram of hepatitis B virus is shown in Figure 4.1. The hepatitis B virus is a member of the *Hepadnaviridae* family, and other very similar viruses in this family cause liver disease in woodchucks, ground squirrels, and ducks. In fact, these animals have served as experimental models for research on human hepatitis B.

The genetic material of hepatitis B virus is a circular strand of DNA. This circular DNA encodes four viral proteins, two of which are structural proteins of the viral particle (Table 4.3). It is important to be familiar with these proteins, especially the hepatitis B surface and core proteins, because detection of these proteins in the blood, or detection of antibodies against them, plays a critical role in diagnosis.

The hepatitis B virus surface antigen (HBsAg) is the "Australia antigen" discovered by Dr. Blumberg. HBsAg is a major

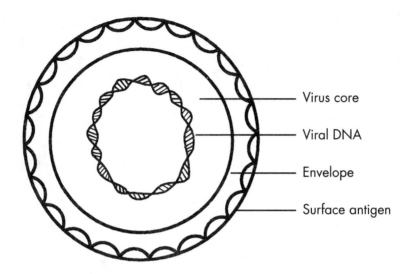

Virus core

Viral DNA

Envelope

Surface antigen

Figure 4.1. *Schematic diagram of the hepatitis B virus.*

The virus contains a core, or nucleocapsid, with which viral DNA is associated. This is surrounded by an envelope that contains the surface antigen.

structural component of the viral particle that is present on its surface. *Testing a patient's blood for circulating hepatitis B surface antigen is presently the single most important test for infection with the hepatitis B virus.*

Hepatitis B core protein (HBcAg) forms the nucleocapsid, or core, of the viral particle and is associated with the viral DNA. Hepatitis B core protein is not readily detectable in the blood of infected individuals but can be seen in the liver cells. If the virus is rapidly replicating in the liver, a smaller form of the hepatitis B core protein can be detected in the infected patient's blood. This form is known as hepatitis Be antigen (HBeAg). Detection of HBeAg in the blood has important clinical significance in the diagnosis of more serious and more highly contagious disease.

Table 4.3. *Proteins of the hepatitis B virus and their functions.*

Protein	Function
Surface antigen (HBsAg)	Structural protein on the surface of the virus. Also circulates as spherical and filamentous aggregates in the blood of infected individuals.
Core antigen (HBcAg)	Core or nucleocapsid of the virus. A shorter form of HBcAg, known as Be antigen (HBeAg), is found in the blood of individuals when the virus is rapidly replicating.
DNA polymerase (pol)	A virally encoded enzyme essential for viral DNA replication.
Protein X	A protein of unclear function; may be involved in carcinogenesis.

Infection with the hepatitis B virus causes both acute and chronic hepatitis. The symptoms and courses of the illness are completely different. The most important determinant for whether hepatitis B virus infection will become chronic is the age at which the individual is infected. About 90 percent of infected newborn babies become chronically infected with hepatitis B virus. About 50 percent of young children who are infected become chronically infected. In adults, only about 5 percent to 10 percent of newly infected individuals become chronically infected.

Some hypothetical case histories are illustrative before discussing acute and chronic hepatitis B and the various ways in which patients can present:

CASE 1. A forty-five-year-old active intravenous heroin user comes to the emergency room complaining of nausea, vomiting, abdominal pain, and yellow eyes. Blood tests show both ALT and AST activity and bilirubin concentration to be elevated. Another blood test detects HBsAg. The patient is admitted to a drug rehabilitation program, and over the next few weeks feels much better. A month later, he is no longer jaundiced and laboratory tests are normal. A repeat test for blood HBsAg is negative.

CASE 2. Another forty-five-year-old intravenous heroin user is brought to the emergency room by ambulance after being found comatose on the street. He is jaundiced. Blood tests indicate elevated ALT and AST activities, elevated bilirubin concentration, prolonged prothrombin time, and detectable HBsAg. He is admitted to the intensive care unit and put on a mechanical ventilator. The coma deepens and he dies.

CASE 3. A twenty-five-year-old woman who was born in China and emigrated to the U.S. has been healthy her entire life. She graduated from college and business school and now works as a securities analyst. She is married and now pregnant for the first time. A routine blood test performed by her obstetrician detects HBsAg in her blood. All other blood tests are normal and she feels fine.

CASE 4. A thirty-nine-year-old homosexual man sees his doctor because he feels tired all the time. Blood tests show elevations in ALT and AST activities. A test for HBsAg is positive. Six months later, blood ALT and AST activities are again elevated and HBsAg is again detected. A blood test for HBeAg is also positive. A liver biopsy shows chronic hepatitis, fibrosis, and cirrhotic nodules.

CASE 5. A sixty-nine-year-old man who was born in Korea has been in good health all his life. He sees a doctor for the first time in more than fifty years because of an inability to fit into his pants and mild abdominal pain. A blood test detects HBsAg. An ultrasound examination shows a shrunken, nodular liver with a mass. Biopsy of the liver mass reveals a hepatocellular carcinoma.

Acute infection with the hepatitis B virus can range from subclinical to fulminant hepatic failure. In newborn babies, acute infection, usually transmitted from the mother at the time of delivery, generally does not cause clinical disease. In younger children, acute infection with hepatitis B virus also does not usually cause clinically apparent disease. In adults, many or most acutely infected individuals develop acute clinical hepatitis that varies in severity.

In most adult cases, acute infection due to hepatitis B virus is moderate and spontaneously resolves. An example is given in case 1 above. Symptoms of hepatitis typically occur between six to fifteen weeks after infection. Symptoms include nausea, vomiting, fever, right upper quadrant abdominal pain, and jaundice. Blood ALT and AST activities are elevated roughly in proportion to the degree of acute inflammation and liver cell death.

Elevations in blood bilirubin concentration and, in more severe cases, prolongation of prothrombin time may also occur. About 2 percent of infected adults develop fulminant hepatic failure. This is what happened to the patient described in case 2. Most of these individuals either die or require emergency liver transplantation. About 90 percent of acutely infected adults, as seen in case 1, have spontaneous resolution of acute hepatitis. The remaining 5 to 10 percent of individuals infected as adults go on to develop chronic hepatitis B, as did the patient in case 4.

Hepatitis B virus infection is the leading cause of chronic liver disease in the world. Most chronically infected individuals are infected as infants or children. Chronic infection can cause various problems. Some chronically infected individuals are clinically classified as *chronic carriers.* Chronic carriers have no clinically apparent liver disease; however, this may be an inaccurate term as some so-called chronic carriers exhibit evidence of hepatitis on liver biopsy. Other individuals chronically infected with hepatitis B virus have clinically apparent chronic hepatitis. Long-standing chronic hepatitis resulting from hepatitis B can lead to cirrhosis. Long-standing hepatitis B infection is also a major risk factor for the development of *hepatocellular carcinoma* or primary liver cancer, which is the number one or two (along with lung cancer) cause of cancer death worldwide.

Chronic carriers are considered to be individuals persistently infected with the hepatitis B virus who do not have clinical evidence of hepatitis. The woman described in case 3 above is an example of a chronic carrier. Chronic carriers have detectable HBsAg in their blood but no signs or symptoms of hepatitis or liver disease. The diagnosis is often made during routine screening of pregnant women, as in case 3, or of blood donors. Typically, blood ALT and AST activities are normal and there is no laboratory evidence of liver damage or dysfunction. The term *chronic carrier* derives from the fact that these individuals have laboratory evidence of hepatitis B virus infection but no clinical or laboratory evidence of liver disease. About 75 percent of chronic carriers will have no evidence of inflammation on liver biopsy and can truly be called "carriers" who do not have evidence of chronic hepatitis. About 25 percent of chronic carriers, however, are not really only "carriers" and will have evidence of inflammation on liver biopsy. These individuals have chronic hepatitis despite normal laboratory tests and no exhibition of symptoms. Some so-called chronic carriers may even have cirrhosis if liver biopsy is performed. Therefore, although almost universally used to describe patients chronically infected with hepatitis B virus and no evidence of liver disease, "chronic carrier" may not technically be a correct description of all such patients. Furthermore, individuals who are defined as chronic carriers can sometimes develop clinically apparent hepatitis at a later time.

Chronic hepatitis that is clinically apparent, as in the hypothetical patient described in case 4, occurs in many individuals chronically infected with the hepatitis B virus. These individuals have detectable serum HBsAg. They may have symptoms of chronic hepatitis including fatigue, depression, loss of appetite, and other nonspecific complaints. Sometimes, the disease is clinically silent and the patient will not have symptoms. Blood tests will usually reveal elevated ALT and AST activities. Sometimes, chronic hepatitis will be diagnosed only by liver biopsy in an individual who is diagnosed clinically as a "chronic carrier."

Individuals with chronic hepatitis B infection, especially those with evidence of ongoing liver inflammation, are at risk of developing cirrhosis over time. Signs and symptoms of cirrhosis may not be apparent and the diagnosis may be made only on liver biopsy. Case 4 describes such an example. Some patients with long-standing chronic hepatitis B may not even come to medical attention until they are suffering from complications of cirrhosis (for examples, see cases 4 and 5).

Individuals with chronic hepatitis B infection, especially those with cirrhosis, are at increased risk for development of hepatocellular carcinoma (primary liver cancer), as exemplified by the hypothetical patient described in case 5. Although relatively rare in the U.S., hepatocellular carcinoma is the number one or number two cause of cancer death in the world, especially in certain Asian and African countries. Individuals with hepatitis B and cirrhosis bear the greatest risk for development of hepatocellular carcinoma. Individuals with hepatitis and no cirrhosis are also at increased risk compared to the general population.

Chronic hepatitis B infection is separated into two distinguishable "states." For simplicity, the best way to distinguish these two states of hepatitis B virus infection is by the presence or absence of hepatitis Be antigen (HBeAg) in blood. In instances where the hepatitis B virus is rapidly replicating, a short form of the hepatitis B core antigen, called HBeAg, is usually detected in the blood. HBeAg is detected in the blood during acute infection, when the virus rapidly replicates, and becomes undetectable as the acute infection resolves. In most cases of chronic infection, HBeAg is not detected because the virus enters a state of low replication and its genetic material integrates into the DNA of infected cells. In some cases of chronic infection, however, the virus maintains a highly replicative "lifestyle" (are viruses alive?) and, in most of these cases, HBeAg will be detected in the blood. In individuals chronically infected with hepatitis B virus, the state of infection can switch from HBeAg-positive (high replication) to HBeAg-negative (low replication) at any time.

The distinction between HBeAg-positive and HBeAg-negative chronic hepatitis B is critical regarding disease severity, prognosis, contagiousness, and treatment. Patients who have HBeAg in their blood usually have more severe clinical disease with a greater amount of inflammation in the liver. They are usually sicker and have more symptoms. The chances of progression to cirrhosis and hepatocellular carcinoma are greater. In addition, *individuals with detectable HBeAg in their blood are highly infectious as high viral replication is associated with the presence of more viral particles in the blood.* At the present time, the main goal of treatment for chronic hepatitis B is to convert a patient who has detectable HBeAg in the blood (a state of high virus replication) to one who does not have detectable HBeAg in the blood (a state of low level virus replication). This change after treatment is associated with a better long-term prognosis.

Individuals with chronic hepatitis B virus infection can spontaneously convert from HBeAg-negative to HBeAg-positive. This is associated with worsening disease severity and prognosis. Paradoxically, conversion from HBeAg-positive to HBeAg-negative, which is associated with a better long-term outlook, is associated with a transient worsening of hepatitis and higher elevations in blood ALT and AST activities. This probably occurs because the immune system attacks the hepatocytes in which the virus is rapidly replicating, causing increased liver inflammation and cell death as infected cells are killed. The "flair" in hepatitis associated with conversion from HBeAg-positive to HBeAg-negative usually resolves with improvement in condition.

One important exception to the rule of HBeAg being detectable in the blood of individuals infected with the hepatitis B virus when the virus is rapidly replicating is infection with mutant forms of hepatitis B virus known as *precore mutants.* Precore mutants of the hepatitis B virus have mutations in their core proteins. As a result, they do not make HBeAg, even when they are rapidly replicating. In precore mutant infection, the presence or absence of HBeAg in the blood is therefore not a determinant of prognosis. Infection with hepatitis B virus precore mutants is relatively uncommon. It may be suspected on clinical grounds, but can be definitively diagnosed only by isolating the virus from the patient and examining its DNA sequence.

Transmission

As many as 300 million individuals throughout the world are chronically infected with the hepatitis B virus, making it the number one worldwide cause of liver disease. The geographic distribution of cases varies tremendously from one part of the world to another. Hepatitis B infection is relatively uncommon in the U.S. and other Western countries. In the U.S., just over one million individuals are chronically infected with hepatitis B virus. On the other hand, hepatitis B infection is endemic in Southeast Asia and sub-Saharan Africa. In countries such as Senegal, Thailand, and parts of China, as many as 25 percent of the population may become infected with hepatitis B virus by early childhood. As a result, liver cancer resulting from chronic hepatitis B virus infection is either the number one or number two cause of cancer death worldwide. The prevalence of infection due to hepatitis B virus in different regions around the world is shown in Figure 4.2.

Hepatitis B virus is transmitted by blood and blood products. It is also transmitted by sex. The virus is also transmitted from mother to newborn baby. The major routes of transmission vary in different parts of the world. In Western countries, including the U.S., intravenous drug use and sex are very important modes of transmission. In other parts of the world where infection is endemic, transmission from mother to newborn is the most important mode of transmission. The major risk factors for transmission of hepatitis B virus are:

- Infected mother to newborn baby
- Blood transfusions (prior to 1970 in developed countries)
- Intravenous drug use

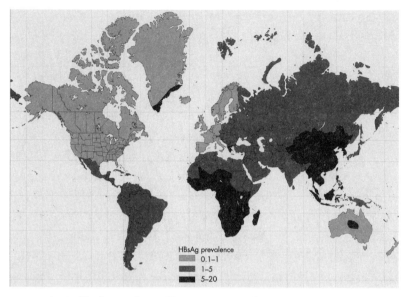

Figure 4.2. *Worldwide prevalence of hepatitis B virus infection.*

The prevalence of infection is extremely high in parts of Asia and Africa.

- Homosexual sex
- Heterosexual sex
- Health care workers exposed to blood
- Infected health care workers to patients (rare)
- Hemodialysis
- Staff of institutions for developmentally challenged
- Men incarcerated in prison (most likely homosexual sex)
- Household contacts of infected individuals

Transmission of hepatitis B virus from mother to fetus may occur either before delivery or by exposure to the mother's blood at the time of delivery. The hepatitis B virus is also present in the breast milk of infected mothers, but a large study has shown that breast feeding is not a major source of transmission of hepatitis B. Some babies of infected mothers who are not infected with the hepatitis B virus at birth become infected during the first few months or first year of life—probably by household exposure to the mother's blood or that of infected brothers or sisters.

A major route of transmission of hepatitis B in the West was transfusion of blood and blood products. Since the association of the "Australia antigen" with serum hepatitis in the 1960s, tremendous efforts have been taken to screen the blood supply and keep it free of hepatitis B virus. In most industrialized countries, the risk of contracting hepatitis B from a blood transfusion is extremely low as donated blood is screened for the presence of the virus. Intravenous drug users and other individuals at high risk for hepatitis B are also excluded from donating blood if they are identified. Although the blood supply is remarkably safe, no screening test is perfect, and the risk of contracting hepatitis B from a transfusion of one unit of blood is approximately 1 in 60,000 to 1 in 100,000 in the U.S. The hepatitis B virus can also be transmitted by organ transplantation but the organ donor's blood is generally tested for hepatitis B virus infection before an organ is used.

Hepatitis B virus can be transmitted by sharing needles. Intravenous drug users frequently share needles to inject heroin or cocaine, and blood is transmitted from one individual to the other via needle. In inner cities in the U.S., intravenous drug use is a major risk factor for hepatitis B. Hepatitis B virus can also be transmitted by tattooing, acupuncture, ear piercing, and piercing of other body parts if unsterilized needles are used.

The hepatitis B virus can also be transmitted by sexual contact. Individuals with multiple sexual partners are at significantly increased risk for hepatitis B. Male homosexuals and female professional sex workers have much higher rates of hepatitis B virus infection than the general population. Patients at sexually transmitted disease clinics also have higher incidences of hepatitis B. Male prisoners are at increased risk for hepatitis B, most likely due to increased rates of unprotected homosexual activities among inmates and also because many are intravenous drug users. In households with an infected individual, the sexual partner runs a higher risk of contracting hepatitis B than from other household contact. Sexual transmission of hepatitis B virus most often occurs by intercourse, either anal or vaginal, as hepatitis B virus can be isolated from semen. The sexual transmission rate from infected women to men is probably less than that from men to women or men to men. Sexual transmission from women to men does occur, however.

Health care workers who are regularly exposed to blood are at increased risk for hepatitis B virus infection. The most likely route of infection is by accidental sticks with needles and other sharp equipment used on infected patients. The hepatitis B virus may also be transmitted by various other pieces of hospital equipment that can contain small quantities of blood, such as unsterilized endoscopes and mechanical ventilators. Hemodialysis is an important route of transmission. Patients with chronic kidney failure who receive hemodialysis are at significantly increased risk for hepatitis B virus infection. There have been sporadic case reports of hepatitis B virus transmission from health care workers to patients. Fortunately, transmission by this route is rare. Most cases have been traced to persistently infected surgeons, dentists, or physicians who perform invasive procedures. Health care workers who transmit the hepatitis B virus to patients are almost always found to be HBeAg-positive upon blood testing.

Staff workers at institutions for the developmentally disabled are also at increased risk for hepatitis B. Hepatitis B virus can most likely be transmitted by biting. This is not uncommon among residents of such institutions. Inapparent exposure to infected blood is probably also relatively common at such institutions.

Household contacts with common objects by infected individuals also increase the risk of contracting hepatitis B. Transmission by blood that is not always obvious occurs among household members, and possible household instruments of transmission include shared razors, toothbrushes, baby bottles, and children's toys. Transmission of hepatitis B virus does not occur by touching, holding hands, kissing, or hugging.

Diagnosis

The first step to diagnose suspected hepatitis B infection, either acute or chronic, is by blood testing. Various blood tests used in the diagnosis of hepatitis B infection are outlined in Table 4.4.

DIAGNOSIS OF ACUTE HEPATITIS B. Hepatitis B surface antigen (HBsAg) in the blood is the most commonly used marker to detect the presence of hepatitis B virus infection. Its detection is a relatively simple procedure in the clinical laboratory. HBsAg is present in the blood early in the course of infection and remains present in the blood during chronic infection. *HBsAg disappears from the blood when infection resolves and its loss means that the patient is cured.*

Antibodies of the IgM class against the hepatitis B core antigen (IgM anti-HBc) are detected in acute infection. They become detectable in the blood shortly after the appearance of HBsAg and remain detectable for a few weeks after HBsAg is lost while the disease is resolving. Testing for IgM anti-HBc is therefore important in a patient who presents late in the course of acute hepatitis B. If IgM anti-HBc is detectable, but HBsAg is not, it indicates that that patient is in the resolution stage of acute hepatitis B.

Antibodies of the IgG class against the hepatitis B core antigen (IgG anti-HBc) are present in the blood of almost all indi-

Table 4.4. *Blood tests for hepatitis B virus infection.*

HBsAg

Present early in infection, remains in chronic infection (if absent, the patient does not have chronic infection). Disappears with resolution of infection.

IgM anti-HBc

Present in acute infection and disappears with resolution.

IgG anti-HBc

Present in individuals chronically infected or in those previously infected. Hence, detection in the absence of HBsAg does not indicate chronic infection.

anti-HBs

Present in previously infected individuals who have cleared the virus from their bodies. Protective against reinfection. Not present in chronically infected individuals. Also induced by vaccination.

HBeAg

Present in patients with very active viral replication. Individuals with chronic infection who are HBeAg-positive are highly infectious and generally have a poorer prognosis.

IgG anti-HBe

Present in patients without high viral replication.

viduals who have been infected with, or possibly exposed to, the virus. These antibodies become detectable in the blood a few months after acute infection, usually after the IgM class antibodies disappear. IgG anti-HBc *persists* in the blood after infection resolves, sometimes for the patient's lifetime. They may be detected in someone with acute infection that is nearly resolved. IgG anti-HBc is not protective against subsequent hepatitis B virus infection.

Individuals with hepatitis B virus infection who clear the virus from their bodies develop antibodies against hepatitis B surface antigen (anti-HBs). If present, these antibodies indicate protection against reinfection. Anti-HBs antibodies are virtually never present in chronically infected individuals who have HBsAg. They are also the type of antibodies induced by vaccination.

The significance of hepatitis Be antigen (HBeAg) has been discussed previously in reference to states of high viral replication versus low viral replication. HBeAg is detectable in the blood of patients with high levels of viral replication. It is present in the blood of individuals with acute infection because, in acute infection, the virus replicates at a high level. Antibodies against HBeAg (IgG anti-HBe) are usually present in the blood of individuals with hepatitis B who do not have HBeAg, that is, those who have low level viral replication.

In individuals with suspected acute hepatitis B virus infection, blood testing for HBsAg, IgM anti-HBc, and anti-HBs should be performed. Acute hepatitis B virus infection is usually suspected in the patient who presents with new onset jaundice and other symptoms including fatigue, right upper quadrant abdominal pain, fever, loss of appetite, nausea, and vomiting. A risk factor for infection may be elicited from the patient's history such as intravenous drug use, an accidental needle stick in a health care worker, or exposure to an infected contact within the past several weeks or months. The presence of HBsAg in blood will indicate acute infection or the continued presence of the virus. The detection of IgM anti-HBc, in the absence of HBsAg, will suggest resolving infection. The presence of anti-HBs will indicate resolution of the disease and that the patient is now immune to future infection. In rare cases, HBsAg and antibodies against it (anti-HBs) can be present at the same time. Such individuals can have complications if these two types of antibodies react with each other in the bloodstream and deposit in the small blood vessels of various organs.

A patient in whom acute hepatitis B virus infection is diagnosed by the presence of HBsAg in the blood should be followed for loss of HBsAg and the development of anti-HBs. In about 90 percent of acutely infected adults, HBsAg will be lost. Most of them will develop HBsAb. In about 5 to 10 percent, however, HBsAg will persist. If HBsAg persists for more than six months after acute infection, the illness is then considered chronic hepatitis B.

DIAGNOSIS OF CHRONIC HEPATITIS B. Chronic hepatitis B is defined as infection with the hepatitis B virus for more than six months. Chronic hepatitis B infection should be suspected in individuals with risk factors (see list on pages 114–115) and individuals from parts of the world where the disease is endemic. Most patients from parts of the world where hepatitis B is endemic were infected as newborn babies or in childhood. A smaller percentage were infected as adults. Most chronically infected individuals in Western countries acquired the disease as adults.

Individuals with chronic hepatitis B infection may have no symptoms (chronic carriers) or have symptoms and clinical evidence of chronic hepatitis, cirrhosis, or even hepatocellular carcinoma. Sometimes, the disease is suspected when elevated ALT and AST activities are detected on routine blood tests or testing for other purposes. *The most important test to establish or exclude chronic hepatitis B is blood testing for HBsAg.*

If HBsAg is detected in the blood, and presumably has been present for more than six months if no recent history of acute hepatitis can be ascertained, chronic hepatitis B virus infection is established. *If HBsAg is not detected in the blood, the individual does not have chronic hepatitis B.* It must be emphasized that, in the absence of HBsAg, the detection of IgG anti-HBc in the blood does not indicate a diagnosis of chronic hepatitis B. This is critical to realize and is a mistake that I have seen many doctors make. *HBsAg must be detected in the blood, or the individual does not have chronic hepatitis B.* In individuals with clinical evidence of chronic hepatitis who do not have detectable blood HBsAg, a search for another cause of hepatitis (e.g., hepatitis C, alcohol, drugs, etc.) should be initiated.

For individuals in whom chronic hepatitis B virus infection is established, that is, those who have had HBsAg in the blood for more than six months, further evaluation is indicated. The blood AST and ALT activities should be checked, as should biochemical tests related to liver function such as albumin concentration, bilirubin concentration, and prothrombin time. If all of these are normal, then the patient is generally considered to be a "chronic carrier." Abnormalities suggest chronic hepatitis and possibly cirrhosis.

Individuals with chronic hepatitis B virus infection and HBsAg should be tested for HBeAg. The presence of serum HBeAg indicates high viral replication, a highly infectious state and possible indication for treatment. The absence of serum HBeAg and/or the presence of anti-HBe suggests a low state of viral replication and a generally better prognosis.

What is the role of liver biopsy in a patient with chronic hepatitis B infection? If any controversy exists, it is probably in individuals who are clinically diagnosed as "chronic carriers." These are patients who have HBsAg in the blood but no symptoms and normal ALT and AST activities. Many liver specialists would say that such individuals do not need liver biopsies. Their argument would be that, at the present time, there is no treatment for such individuals and they *most likely* will have minimal or no liver inflammation. This is all true. However, many liver specialists will advocate liver biopsy for such patients. Although most chronic carriers will have normal liver biopsies, about 25 percent of chronic carriers will have inflammation on liver biopsy and a few will even have cirrhosis. Even if you knew this, there are no recommended treatment interventions at the present time for those individuals who do not have detectable blood HBeAg.

In the end, the decision to perform a liver biopsy on a patient diagnosed as a hepatitis B virus "chronic carrier" probably should depend upon the desire of the patient, and doctor, to want to better assess the state of the patient's liver. Some patients will want to know if they have cirrhosis or ongoing inflammation, which would be correlated with a poorer prognosis than no inflammation or cirrhosis. Some patients do not want to know. The final decision to perform liver biopsy in a clinically diagnosed hepatitis B "chronic carrier" therefore depends upon the desire to know as much as possible about prognosis.

Most liver specialists will probably agree that their patients with chronic hepatitis B who exhibit clinical and/or laboratory evidence of hepatitis should have liver biopsies if there are no contraindications. Nonetheless, there are no recommended treatment options at this time for patients who do not have detectable HBeAg in the blood. The chance of having cirrhosis is much greater in a patient with hepatitis B infection and ongoing hepatitis than in a chronic carrier without evidence of hepatitis, however. And in many cases, only a liver biopsy can definitely establish the presence of cirrhosis.

Patients with chronic hepatitis B and detectable HBeAg in blood should have liver biopsies if there are no contraindications. Most of these patients will have clinical and/or laboratory evidence of hepatitis. The degree of inflammation and, in most cases, the presence or absence of cirrhosis can be established only by examination of the liver biopsy. These patients are also candidates for treatment and, before any treatment is considered, a diagnosis should be confirmed.

Treatment

At present, the U.S. Food and Drug Administration (FDA) has approved two drugs for the treatment of chronic hepatitis B: recombinant interferon alpha-2b (Intron-A) and lamivudine (Epivir-HBV). Other preparations of interferon alpha and other type I interferons may also be equally effective. They have not yet been approved for this indication, however. It is not clear at this time whether to use interferon alpha-2b first followed by lamivudine if a patient does not respond to interferon, to use lamivudine first, or use a combination of both. It is also not known if certain subgroups of patients will have better results with one drug or the other. These questions will likely be answered over the next few years. Here, each of these drugs will be discussed separately. The choice to use one or the other depends upon the specific patient and doctor.

Which patients with hepatitis B should be considered for treatment? The following criteria should be considered:

- Chronic hepatitis B (infection lasting longer than six months) with detectable serum HBsAg
- Replicative infection with detectable serum HBeAg
- No ascites, encephalopathy, and/or bleeding esophageal varices
- Normal, stable serum albumin concentration

- Normal or almost normal serum bilirubin concentration
- Prothrombin time no more than three seconds greater than a normal control

Patients should first have chronic hepatitis B (longer than six months with infection) documented by the presence of HBsAg in their blood. To be eligible for treatment, patients should have replicative hepatitis B infection, that is, they should have detectable HBeAg in their blood. At this time, treatment is *not* recommended for patients without detectable HBeAg. Prior to commencing treatment, patients with HBeAg-positive chronic hepatitis B should have a liver biopsy to confirm the diagnosis. Patients who have clinical complications of cirrhosis, such as ascites, encephalopathy, and/or bleeding esophageal varices, should probably not be treated, except in research studies. Patients with biochemical evidence of compromised liver function, including low blood albumin concentration, elevated bilirubin concentration, or prolonged prothrombin time more than three seconds greater than a control, should probably not be treated. Patients with significantly low platelet counts, low white blood counts, or significant anemia should probably not receive interferon alpha-2b; however, the exact cutoff values for exclusion are not agreed upon by all doctors. Patients with hypothyroidism, hyperthyroidism, or diabetes mellitus and poorly controlled blood sugars should not be treated with interferon alpha-2b until these conditions are medically controlled.

INTERFERON ALPHA-2B. Patients with HBeAg-positive chronic hepatitis B should be treated with a dose of 5 million units of interferon alpha-2b every day. An alternative regimen is 10 million units three times a week. Interferon alpha-2b comes either as a powder that must be mixed with sterile water before use, or as an already mixed solution. The powder and premixed solutions are stable if stored in the refrigerator. Interferon alpha-2b is administered by subcutaneous (under the skin) or intramuscular (into the muscle) injections. Most patients self-administer injections with small syringes and needles similar to those used by diabetics to inject insulin. Recently, the manufacturer has started marketing an "injection pen" to facilitate injections. Most people choose to inject the interferon into the thigh; however, other areas such as the abdomen can also be injected. Patients should obtain brief training from a doctor or nurse before beginning self-injections.

Interferon alpha-2b treatment for HBeAg-positive chronic hepatitis B lasts sixteen weeks. Because low blood counts are a side effect of interferon alpha-2b treatment, patients should have their blood drawn and complete blood counts and platelet counts checked at 1, 2, 4, 8, 12, and 16 weeks after treatment has begun. ALT activity, bilirubin concentration, and albumin concentration should also be checked periodically during therapy. Patients should probably be seen by their doctors, or a nurse, at least once a month during treatment and instructed to contact their doctor if they experience side effects.

At the dosage levels used to treat hepatitis B, the most common and potentially serious side effects of interferon alpha-2b are low neutrophil counts and low platelet counts. Neutrophils, also called granulocytes, are a particular type of white blood cell important in fighting bacterial infections. Platelets are tiny blood cells involved in clotting that may also be low in individuals with cirrhosis. As mentioned above, patients should have their blood counts monitored during treatment with interferon alpha-2b. If the neutrophil count falls below 750 cells per cubic millimeter of blood or the platelet count falls below 50,000 cells per cubic millimeter of blood, the daily dose can be cut in half until these values rise above these levels. If the neutrophil count falls below 500 cells per cubic millimeter of blood or the platelet count below 30,000 cells per cubic millimeter of blood, interferon alpha-2b therapy should (probably) be discontinued and (possibly) resumed only when the counts return to their baseline values.

There are *many* other side effects of interferon alpha therapy beside low blood counts. The most common is development of flu-like symptoms. These can be quite disabling and include fever, cold sweats, shaking chills, muscle aches and pains, and joint aches and pains. Flu-like symptoms are usually worse near the start of treatment and less common later in the course of therapy. To help tolerate mild to moderate flu-like symptoms, I generally recommend that patients inject the interferon about an hour before going to sleep and take acetaminophen just before injecting the interferon. The acetaminophen will provide some relief from symptoms and, if taken at bedtime, possibly help the patient to sleep through the side effects. Flu-like symptoms rarely require stopping treatment, but on occasion they are so intolerable that there is no other option.

Interferon alpha treatment can aggravate diabetes mellitus and thyroid disorders. Patients with diabetes mellitus who are treated with interferon alpha should carefully monitor their blood sugars. Patients with thyroid disease, and possibly all treated patients, should have blood tests for thyroid function checked periodically during treatment. Significant abnormalities in blood sugar or thyroid tests may necessitate stopping treatment.

Nervous system and psychiatric problems have been reported in individuals receiving interferon alpha-2b. Tingling in the hands, feet, arms, and legs are the most common nervous system side effect. Depression, irritability, confusion, nervousness, impaired concentration, anxiety, and insomnia have all occurred in individuals taking interferon alpha-2b. Sometimes these psychiatric problems are so severe that treatment must be stopped. Severe depression has occurred in individuals taking interferon and suicides have been reported. Patients with serious preexisting depression or other psychiatric disorders probably should not be treated with interferon alpha, and if severe depression develops, the drug should be discontinued immediately and the patient closely followed and referred to a psychiatrist as necessary.

Virtually every complaint has been reported by patients receiving interferon alpha-2b. Other, more frequent side effects, which are usually not severe, include fever, rash, headache, muscle aches, fatigue, back pain, dry mouth, nausea, diarrhea, and inflammation at the injection site. Rare patients have what appear to be allergic reactions to interferon alpha, and the drug must be discontinued if these occur. Despite numerous side effects, interferon alpha-2b therapy is rather safe if patients are monitored closely. Most patients complete the recommended course of therapy.

What are the goals of interferon alpha-2b therapy for chronic hepatitis B? The primary goals are to decrease liver inflammation (reduced blood ALT activity is an approximate marker) and change the infection from replicative (blood HBeAg-positive) to non-replicative (blood HBeAg-negative). Another goal is cure or loss of HBsAg from blood. ALT activity, HBsAg, and HBeAg should be checked by blood testing at the end of therapy, one month after therapy, and six months after therapy. Many patients will not have a detectable response during treatment but will have detectable responses between one and six months after stopping therapy. Many individuals with chronic hepatitis B who are treated with interferon alpha-2b have a lowering of blood ALT activities after treatment. In studies having the best results, about 40 percent of treated patients lose HBeAg. In other studies, the loss rates of HBeAg from the blood have been around 20 percent. Patients who lose

HBeAg after interferon alpha treatment have been shown to have a better prognosis, probably because the degree of liver inflammation is decreased and the progression to cirrhosis is slowed significantly.

A low percentage of patients with HBeAg-positive chronic hepatitis B who are treated with interferon alpha-2b lose HBsAg from the blood and may be considered to be completely cured. Although the loss rate of HBsAg after interferon treatment is significantly greater than what occurs spontaneously without treatment, it is still rather low. The best studies have shown rates of loss of HBsAg of only 10 percent, and most studies show rates of only a few percent.

Some patients treated with chronic hepatitis B will have a paradoxical flare in liver inflammation as indicated by an elevation in blood ALT activity during treatment with interferon alpha. This flare is often associated with loss of HBeAg and results from the immune system being stimulated to destroy the virus-infected liver cells. Therefore, if a sudden rise in ALT activity occurs during interferon alpha-2b treatment in an individual with chronic hepatitis B, therapy should be continued unless evidence of worsening liver *function* or failure is detected.

Who is likely to respond to treatment with interferon alpha-2b? A shorter duration of infection correlates to a better chance of response. Individuals from countries where hepatitis B virus infection is endemic, and were likely infected at birth or in early childhood, are therefore less likely to respond to interferon alpha-2b. People infected as adults and who have been infected for less than three years usually have the best response. Younger patients are more likely to respond than older patients. Patients without cirrhosis will respond more often than those with cirrhosis; however, patients with greater inflammation on biopsy may surprisingly respond better than those with minimal inflammation.

LAMIVUDINE. Lamivudine is a molecule that looks like a building block of DNA. Its mechanism of action is to inhibit the DNA polymerase of the hepatitis B virus. The activity of this enzyme is essential for replication of the virus. Lamivudine belongs to the class of drugs known as nucleoside analogues. Lamivudine (also known as 3TC) is also approved for another indication: the treatment of human immunodeficiency virus (HIV) infection. HIV has a DNA polymerase called reverse transcriptase that is inhibited by lamivudine (as well as other drugs, the most famous of which is probably AZT). Similarly, lamivudine inhibits the hepatitis B virus DNA polymerase. For the treatment of chronic hepatitis B, the dose is 100 mg of lamivudine a day. The daily dose for HIV infection is higher.

Large clinical studies indicate that lamivudine works better than a placebo (dummy drug) in reducing liver inflammation measured on biopsy and in causing a loss of serum HBeAg from blood. One preliminary study suggested that lamivudine was equally effective as interferon alpha-2b in bringing about a loss of HBeAg in a head-to-head comparison. Most studies have examined treatment for one year, but the most effective duration of treatment has not been firmly established. The safety of treatment beyond one year has also not been established.

Lamivudine is generally well tolerated in patients with chronic hepatitis B. In clinical trials, the most common adverse events were ear, nose, and throat infections, plus fatigue and headache. These were reported by approximately one-fifth to one-quarter of patients. More serious adverse events were very unusual.

A major advantage of lamivudine compared to interferon alpha-2b is that it is administered orally. One possible drawback is that liver inflammation may recur after the drug is discontinued (in most studies, lamivudine was administered for up to one year). Another drawback is that the hepatitis B virus can mutate and become resistant to lamivudine during treatment. It is associated with a specific type of mutation in the viral gene (pol) that encodes the DNA polymerase. Resistance is seen in about 10 to 20 percent of treated patients. If the virus becomes resistant to lamivudine, blood ALT and AST activities may rise and the concentration of hepatitis B virus DNA in the blood becomes elevated if it is measured. If lamivudine is stopped, the mutant virus appears to die out and a nonmutant virus replaces it in the blood. Fortunately, the onset of resistance does not appear to be associated with severe liver disease.

The final data on lamivudine are not yet in, but it is very simple to administer and appears very safe. Its use is associated with improvements in liver inflammation and, in some patients, loss of detectable HBeAg from the blood indicating lower viral replication and a better prognosis. Studies are now under way to examine combination and sequential therapy with lamivudine and interferon alpha-2b for patients with chronic hepatitis B.

OTHER DRUGS IN THE NEAR FUTURE? Several other drugs are in clinical trials for the treatment of chronic hepatitis B. Like interferon alpha-2b and lamivudine, most of these drugs will probably be for patients with high viral replication and detectable HBeAg in blood. Most of the drugs presently being used in early clinical trials, like lamivudine, are nucleoside analogues that inhibit the hepatitis B virus DNA polymerase. Having several DNA polymerase inhibitors available will likely prove a major advantage in treatment as mutations that make the virus resistant to one may not make it resistant to another. In the not-too-distant future, one can imagine treatment for chronic hepatitis B with two or more DNA polymerase inhibitors and possibly another drug such as interferon alpha.

Perhaps the greatest challenge in the treatment of chronic hepatitis B infection are patients with low levels of viral replication, that is, those without detectable HBeAg in the blood. This constitutes the majority of the world's hepatitis B patients.

Most available treatments attack the replicating virus. But because the viral genetic material is integrated into the host cell DNA when replication is very low, it is unclear exactly how to attack the virus in this state. Future research will undoubtedly provide new possibilities, but effective treatments for HBeAg-negative chronic hepatitis B and chronic carriers will probably not be available in the near future.

Medical follow-up and cancer screening

Patients with chronic hepatitis B infection should have regular medical checkups whether or not they are candidates for treatment. Even chronic carriers should see their doctor regularly. If a patient has clinically apparent chronic hepatitis B for many years without significant clinical changes, that patient should probably see a doctor at least once every twelve months. The same should probably hold true for chronic carriers. A physical examination should be performed to ensure there are no signs of cirrhosis. Blood tests should also be taken periodically. Individuals with cirrhosis caused by chronic hepatitis B may have to be seen more frequently for changes in their condition and referral to a liver transplantation center if complications become difficult to control, or if blood tests indicate progressive liver dysfunction.

An important aspect of follow-up care for patients chronically infected with hepatitis B virus is screening for hepatocellular carcinoma. Individuals with chronic hepatitis B infection, especially those with cirrhosis, are at a significantly increased risk for development of hepatocellular carcinoma (primary liver cancer). Although strict guidelines have not been established regarding testing frequency, and little to no data exist on overall efficacy and cost-effectiveness, it is generally agreed that patients with chronic hepatitis B virus infection should have periodic screening for liver cancer. These patients should have periodic ultrasound studies to check for small liver masses. In addition, blood should periodically be tested for alpha-fetoprotein, which is a marker for hepatocellular carcinoma. Most liver specialists would probably perform such screenings approximately once a year in individuals with known cirrhosis. Even individuals without known cirrhosis should probably be periodically screened, including chronic carriers once they reach age forty. Again, good data on the efficacy and cost effectiveness of this type of screening do not exist and it is up to the individual doctor's judgment to determine how frequently "periodic" cancer screening should be performed.

Hepatitis B virus–hepatitis C virus–human immunodeficiency virus co-infection

The modes of transmission of hepatitis B virus are quite similar to those for hepatitis C virus and human immunodeficiency virus (HIV). Hence, it is not unusual for individuals to be infected with any two, or even all three, of these viruses at the same time. A detailed discussion of all the possible diagnostic and treatment options for co-infected patients is beyond the scope of this book, and a lot depends upon the particular case and the doctor's judgment. In general, patients with HIV infection but a healthy immune system (normal CD4 or "T-cell" counts) and no complications of AIDS, who have hepatitis B infection, should probably be treated just like patients without HIV infection. Equally aggressive diagnostic procedures and treatments should probably be used if there are no contraindications. In individuals with low CD4 counts or with AIDS, a less aggressive approach to hepatitis B may be taken as other problems may be more immediate. Again, the approach to such patients depends upon the individual case and the doctor's judgment.

For patients with both chronic hepatitis B virus and hepatitis C virus infection, both diseases should be approached together. Many of the diagnostic and treatment considerations are similar to both diseases. Patients with HBeAg-positive hepatitis B, who also have chronic hepatitis C and are candidates for interferon alpha treatment, should probably be treated first at the dose used to treat hepatitis B, and subsequently at the recommended dose and duration for hepatitis C.

Prevention

Hepatitis B is a contagious disease. All individuals infected with hepatitis B virus are potentially contagious. Those who have detectable HBeAg in the blood are especially contagious.

Certain commonsense preventive measures can be used to curtail the spread of hepatitis B among individuals who are not immune. Sexually promiscuous individuals, as well as individuals who do not know much about their single sex partner, should use condoms. Condoms should also be used in sexual relationships if one partner is known to be infected with the hepatitis B virus and the other is not immune. Those living in a household with a hepatitis B virus-infected individual should exhibit caution by avoiding contact with blood, some of which may not be readily apparent. For example, they should not share razors, toothbrushes, or similar items. Caution should be used in tending to injured individuals who are bleeding. In hospitals and doctor's offices, extreme caution should be used in drawing blood and in properly disposing of needles and surgical instruments.

Individuals not immune to hepatitis B infection (those who do not have anti-HBs) who are accidentally exposed to contaminated blood, or have sex with an infected individual, can receive passive immunization with hepatitis B immune globulin (HBIG). HBIG is a preparation of antibodies pooled from the blood of many individuals who are immune to hepatitis B. The antibodies are sterilized so that other viruses are not spread with the immune globulin preparations. HBIG should be given by injection soon after contact, at most within thirty days, to prevent hepatitis B in exposed individuals.

The hepatitis B virus can be transmitted from a pregnant woman to her newborn baby. All pregnant women should be screened for HBsAg in their blood. If it is detected, the newborn should be given HBIG followed by a vaccination series (see below) beginning one week after birth. Several studies suggest that this will significantly decrease the chance of the baby becoming chronically infected with hepatitis B virus.

For several years, effective vaccines against hepatitis B virus have been available. Most current preparations are of recombinant hepatitis B surface antigen manufactured using recombinant DNA technology. Three shots are needed in most individuals to assure long-term immunity. After the initial shot of vaccine, a second shot is given one month later and a third six months later. The large majority of individuals respond to three shots with the development of HBsAb. Elderly individuals, or individuals with chronic diseases, are less likely to respond.

Who should be vaccinated for hepatitis B? At the present time, universal vaccination is recommended for all children. For adults, those who are at high risk of exposure to hepatitis B virus should be vaccinated. This would include health care workers, household members living with an individual with hepatitis B, sexual partners of individuals with chronic hepatitis B, and perhaps all sexually promiscuous individuals. People from Western countries who will reside for extended periods of time in parts of the world where hepatitis B virus infection is endemic should also be vaccinated.

All available scientific data indicate that the hepatitis B vaccines presently in use are extremely safe. Some press reports have focused on a few individuals claiming to have developed "autoimmune disorders" after receiving hepatitis B vaccines. There are no laboratory studies indicating that hepatitis B vaccines can induce such diseases and no forward-looking or case-controlled studies demonstrating that people who have received hepatitis B vaccines have a higher incidence of any diseases compared to those not vaccinated. Such studies, in fact, indicate that there are less diseases, namely hepatitis B and liver cancer, in vaccinated individuals. All of the claims that have so far appeared in the press that claim hepatitis B vaccine may cause "autoimmune disorders" are based on isolated, retrospective (backward-looking) reports that may be coincidental, and do not demonstrate cause and effect. Claims such as these should *not* be considered as scientific evidence.

Theoretically, hepatitis B should be a very rare disease and ultimately eradicated from the globe because effective vaccines are available. In a landmark study in Taiwan, it was demonstrated that universal vaccination against hepatitis B virus led to a reduction in primary liver cancer. Imagine a vaccine that prevents one of the most common causes of cancer death in the world! Well, it really is here! However, socioeconomic and political realities make it difficult to provide hepatitis B vaccines to individuals in the parts of the world where it is needed most. Sadly, hepatitis B will likely be with us for a long time and primary liver cancer will continue to be a leading cause of cancer death worldwide.

Hepatitis C

Definition and symptoms

The discovery of hepatitis C virus in 1989 revolutionized the approach to patients with liver disease, especially in the U.S., Canada, and Europe. Around that same time, interferon alpha was shown to be an effective treatment for what was formerly called "non-A, non-B" hepatitis. As a result of this research, millions of individuals with liver disease were given a diagnosis and offered treatment that previously did not even have a name associated with the diagnosis. In addition, numerous gastroenterologists and other physicians decided that they would now be hepatologists (liver specialists).

Before discussing hepatitis C, it is worthwhile to provide a description of the virus that causes it. Only what I consider to be the essential issues necessary to understand the disease hepatitis C are discussed. The essentials of viral structure and function are discussed and additional details are included only in figures for completeness. Truly interested readers can find additional information in the other sources listed in Appendix B.

The hepatitis C virus was discovered in 1989 by workers at the biotechnology company Chiron Corporation. Its discovery relied entirely on the discipline of molecular biology. Nobody has conclusively seen the hepatitis C virus under an electron microscope, and its existence is based entirely on the cloning of its genetic material. Prior to discovery of the hepatitis C virus, a type of infectious hepatitis was referred to as "non-A, non-B" hepatitis. Individuals with this disease had clinical or laboratory evidence of hepatitis without evidence of hepatitis A or hepatitis B virus infection. Evidence based on transmission patterns suggested that non-A, non-B hepatitis was caused by an unidentified virus. Non-A, non-B hepatitis was observed in patients after they had received blood transfusions. It was also commonly seen in intravenous drug users. Furthermore, blood from individuals with non-A, non-B hepatitis caused hepatitis if injected into chimpanzees, and blood from one infected chimpanzee could transmit hepatitis to another chimpanzee. These findings indicated that another human hepatotropic virus (or viruses) was a significant cause of liver disease.

The creative approach used by workers at Chiron that led to the identification of a new human hepatitis is outlined in Figure 4.3. After identifying the virus using techniques from molecular biology, these investigators and their collaborators demonstrated what was responsible for at least 85 percent of what was then diagnosed as non-A, non-B hepatitis. Their results were published in two papers in the journal *Science* in 1989. The following year, Chiron investigators as well as several other groups of scientists used the partial genetic sequence information to isolate and sequence the complete genetic material of the then-novel hepatitis C virus.

The genetic material of hepatitis C is RNA. Based on sequence similarity, it is a member of the Flaviviridae family of viruses. Viral RNA encodes a large protein that is processed in infected host cells into several smaller structural and nonstructural proteins. This is illustrated in Figure 4.4.

It is not important to remember the names and functions of all the hepatitis C viral proteins. For those who are interested, they are briefly described in Table 4.5. What is important for everyone to remember is that detection of antibodies against these proteins in the blood of infected individuals plays a critical role in diagnosis and screening of the common blood supply. Some of these proteins are also targets of attack for novel drugs that are in development to treat hepatitis C.

Although a few reports have been published in which investigators claimed to have seen the hepatitis C virus with an electron microscope, no one has yet provided conclusive proof. The presumed structure of hepatitis C is inferred from structures of proteins encoded by its genetic material and comparison to other related viruses. The size of the virus is also estimated by passing infectious blood through filters before it is injected into chimpanzees to determine if they develop hepatitis. A schematic

Infect chimpanzees with blood from patients with
post-transfusion non-A, non-B hepatitis

↓

Extract DNA and RNA, some presumably of the putative
hepatitis C virus, from serum of infected chimpanzees

↓

Construct DNA library from DNA and RNA
reverse transcribed to complementary DNA

↓

Express proteins encoded by DNA in the library in bacteria,
some of which are encoded by viral DNA or complementary DNA

↓

Screen bacteria expressing proteins with antibodies from
blood of a patient with non-A, non-B hepatitis that presumably
contains antibodies against the putative hepatitis C virus

↓

Purify DNA clones from bacteria expressing proteins
recognized by antibodies in the patient's blood

↓

Isolate and sequence DNA that corresponds to a portion
of the putative hepatitis virus gene (actually complementary
DNA copy of a portion of the viral RNA genome)

↓

Use this fragment to isolate the rest of the viral genome

Figure 4.3. *Strategy used to identify the hepatitis C virus.*

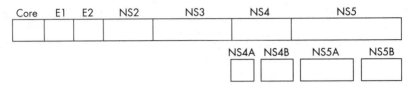

Figure 4.4. *A schematic diagram showing the large protein encoded by the hepatitis C viral RNA molecule and smaller proteins to which it is processed in infected cells.*

The small proteins core, E1, and E2 are structural proteins of the viral particle. The proteins NS2, NS3, NS4A, NS4B, NS5A, and NS5B are not present in the mature virus but are expressed in infected cells. They are essential for viral replication and may have other functions in infected liver cells (see Table 4.5).

diagram of the presumed structure of the hepatitis C virus is shown in Figure 4.5.

Two important issues in hepatitis C virology are those of *genotype* and *quasispecies*. Many liver specialists are determining the genotype of the infecting hepatitis C virus as a matter of routine, and many patients have questions about this. In brief, hepatitis C viruses isolated from different patients show differences in their genetic material. These differences may cause changes in the structures of the encoded proteins. Viral isolates that have significant degrees of dissimilarity belong to different genotypes. There are six major hepatitis C virus genotypes. In the most commonly used current nomenclature, they are referred to as genotypes one though six. There are some sub-genotypes within the six major genotypes identified using letters, for example, 1a and 1b.

Many clinical studies suggest that infection with different hepatitis C virus genotypes may have different clinical consequences. Genotypes 1a and 1b, the most common found in the U.S., have been associated with more aggressive disease and a

Table 4.5. *The proteins of hepatitis C virus.*

Protein	Function
Structural proteins	
Core	Forms the viral particle nucleocapsid or core; may have other effects when expressed in host cells such as regulating apoptosis (cell death) and inhibiting cell protein synthesis
E1	Protein of the envelope
E2	Protein of the envelope
P7	Possible envelope protein
Nonstructural proteins	
NS2	A protease that cleaves the viral polyprotein at a specific site
NS3	A protease that cleaves the viral polyprotein at specific sites and an RNA-helicase that can unwind the viral RNA in cells
NS4A	A cofactor necessary for the NS3 protease
NS4B	Function unknown
NS5A	Function not entirely clear but plays some role in determining sensitivity of viral infection to interferon
NS5B	RNA-polymerase necessary to replicate the viral RNA

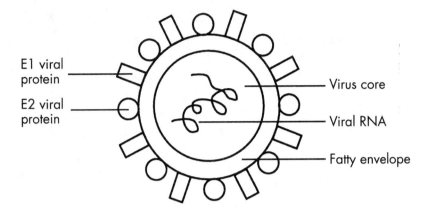

E1 viral protein

E2 viral protein

Virus core

Viral RNA

Fatty envelope

Figure 4.5. *A schematic diagram of the hepatitis C virus.*

The virus contains a single RNA molecule associated with a nucleo-capsid or core in its center. This is surrounded by a fatty envelope that contains two viral proteins—E1 and E2.

greater likelihood of progression to cirrhosis. Infection with non-type 1 genotypes has been associated with a better prognosis. Several studies also suggest that patients infected with genotypes 1a and 1b are less likely to respond to treatment. Although none of the studies on hepatitis C virus genotype and its correlation to clinical disease is absolutely conclusive, most investigators feel that individuals infected with genotypes 1a or 1b will be less likely to respond to treatment with interferon alpha. How determination of genotype in a specific patient should be used to guide treatment, however, has not been clearly established.

Strains of the hepatitis C virus with more subtle differences that may result from either one or several spontaneous mutations are known as quasispecies. The concept of quasispecies may seem like molecular esoterica to the average patient; it indeed may be of clinical relevance, however. Quasispecies represent a way in which the virus changes to avoid being eliminated by the immune system. The emergence of hepatitis C virus quasispecies in an individual with hepatitis C may be associated with more aggressive disease and poor response to treatment. At the present time, quasispecies cannot be determined in commercial laboratories. Their detection requires specialized research procedures.

The hepatitis C virus causes both acute and chronic hepatitis. By far the major concern about being infected with the hepatitis C virus is the development of chronic hepatitis. Acute infection with the hepatitis C virus usually is not associated with symptoms and usually goes undiagnosed. *Acute infection with the hepatitis C virus usually does not cause clinically apparent disease.* Most people who are chronically infected cannot recall an acute episode of jaundice or liver disease. Some may have nonspecific symptoms at the time of infection but never associate them with liver disease. In some cases, however, infection with the hepatitis C virus does cause acute disease. Rare cases of fulminant hepatic failure caused by acute hepatitis C virus infection have been reported and convincingly demonstrated. Although acute hepatitis caused by the hepatitis C virus should always be suspected in an individual with new, sudden onset liver disease, it usually does not turn out to be the cause.

The major concern about hepatitis C virus is that infection becomes chronic in the large majority of cases. It is estimated that, of all people infected with the hepatitis C virus, 85 percent become chronically infected. This appears to be the case in adults and probably in children, too. Although acute infection is usually not accompanied by apparent disease, once the virus enters an individual's body, it has a very high chance of staying there and replicating in the liver during the person's lifetime.

Chronic hepatitis C has been referred to by some as a "silent killer." Perhaps this term is a bit alarmist as only a minority of patients chronically infected with the hepatitis C virus die as a result. There is some accuracy to this term, however. Acute infection with hepatitis C virus is almost always silent and patients almost never remember how they caught the disease. *Once a person is chronically infected with the hepatitis C virus, the symptoms of chronic hepatitis are often not present or are so nonspecific that the diagnosis is not readily made.*

Most patients with chronic hepatitis C have no symptoms or only nonthreatening symptoms such as tiredness, lack of energy, mild depression, and mild loss of appetite. In a sense, the disease is silent. Unless a history of risk factor is elucidated—for example, past intravenous drug use or blood transfusion prior to 1990—the doctor usually does not suspect hepatitis C upon first seeing a patient. The disease is often first suspected when routine blood tests are performed. Mild to moderate elevations in blood ALT and AST activities are frequently detected that suggest chronic hepatitis. If alcohol abuse is not in the differential diagnosis, hepatitis C is the most likely cause, at least in the U.S. Even if the patient is a moderate to heavy alcohol drinker, chronic hepatitis C is still a possibility as alcohol and chronic hepatitis C are often diagnosed together. This may be due to the combination of viral hepatitis and even moderate alcohol use, which is more likely to cause liver disease than either condition alone. Hence, patients with both diseases may be more likely to seek medical attention for liver problems.

What is the course of disease in a chronic hepatitis C patient? The big problem for physicians and patients is that its course is extremely variable and usually cannot be predicted in a specific case. Some patients will have mild, low-grade hepatitis for life and never develop complications of liver disease. Some patients will develop cirrhosis several years after infection while others will *never* exhibit symptoms during many years of infection and see a doctor later in life with clinical evidence of cirrhosis. A few hypothetical case histories are illustrative.

CASE 1. A forty-year-old woman who is very healthy donates blood. She is told that she has antibodies against the hepatitis C virus. She sees a doctor who conducts a normal physical examination with completely normal blood tests, including normal ALT and AST activities. Upon questioning her mother, the patient discovers that she received a blood transfusion as a baby. A reverse transcription-polymerase chain reaction test detects low levels of hepatitis C virus RNA in her blood. A liver biopsy shows an essentially normal liver.

CASE 2. A thirty-nine-year-old man who works as an investment banker is refused life insurance because of "abnormal liver function tests." He routinely works twelve- to fifteen-hour days in a stressful job and jogs and plays tennis regularly. He says that he has never felt better in his life. In college, he experimented only a few times with intravenous drugs but has not used any in twenty years. His doctor finds that a test for antibodies against the hepatitis C virus is positive and a liver biopsy shows moderate liver inflammation with fibrosis (scarring) progressing to cirrhosis.

CASE 3. A fifty-five-year-old woman who works as a nurse remembers sticking herself with a needle about five years ago. She paid little attention to this accident at the time. She feels chronically tired and has mild swelling in her abdomen and ankles and yellowing in the whites of her eyes. She sends off some of her blood to the laboratory and finds elevated ALT and AST activities, a low albumin concentration, and slightly prolonged prothrombin time. She sees a doctor who performs a liver biopsy that indicates cirrhosis.

CASE 4. A seventy-four-year-old woman presents to her doctor with swelling of the abdomen, swollen ankles, and some pain in her abdomen. She has never consumed alcohol. When she was thirty-four years old she had a hysterectomy and needed a blood transfusion because of extensive bleeding during surgery. She was an active, healthy woman for the next forty years with few visits to doctors. Physical examination now reveals ascites, edema, and jaundice. Blood tests show normal ALT and AST activities, low albumin concentration, elevated bilirubin concentration, and prolonged prothrombin time. An ultrasound shows ascites and a shrunken, nodular liver consistent with cirrhosis with a mass very typical for hepatocellular carcinoma. A blood test for antibodies against the hepatitis C virus is positive.

These four cases demonstrate the wide variety of presentations of chronic hepatitis C. In some cases, it is a relatively benign disease, in others a "silent killer," and in still others something in between. The patient described in case 1 has been infected with the hepatitis C virus for forty years but is completely healthy and has a liver biopsy with no evidence of chronic hepatitis. She will probably not suffer any consequences of liver disease in her lifetime and would never have known that she had a chronic hepatitis C virus infection if she had not donated blood. There are millions of people like this around the world. They are chronically infected with hepatitis C, will probably never know it, and will probably never get sick from it. In such cases, the disease is clearly "silent" but not a "killer."

The patient described in case 2 is typical. He was infected with the hepatitis C virus twenty years earlier by experimenting with intravenous drugs. He has never used drugs since and is now a wealthy and successful man. He finds out about possible liver disease through a life insurance examination and is diagnosed with hepatitis C by his doctor. However, he is less fortunate than the patient in case 1 because, after twenty years of hepatitis C virus infection, this patient already has evidence on liver biopsy that he is developing cirrhosis. In his case, the hepatitis C virus may indeed be behaving like a "silent killer." However, the infection may have been detected early enough so that treatment can prove beneficial. He may or may not develop cirrhosis and complications in later years.

The patient described in case 3 represents a less common but possible course of hepatitis C infection. She was infected only five years earlier and already has cirrhosis and clinical complications. The hepatitis C virus usually does not cause such rapid progression of liver disease but it is certainly capable of doing so. Here, the virus is also acting as a "killer," but it is less silent. It may be too late for treatment to prevent progression of this woman's liver disease. Fortunately, liver transplantation may stop the virus from acting as a "killer" in her case.

The hypothetical patient described in case 4 manifests the real "silent killer" aspect of the hepatitis C virus. She was infected for forty years with the virus and never knew it. The diagnosis of chronic hepatitis C was not made until she had advanced cirrhosis and primary liver cancer. This otherwise healthy woman will probably die of liver disease relatively soon after diagnosis.

How many patients infected with hepatitis C virus will be like the patient in case 1? How many like the less fortunate patients such as those in cases 2 through 4? The available data do not permit these questions to be answered precisely, but some estimates can be provided.

Of all the patients who are diagnosed by doctors, most are probably similar to the patient in case 2. Chronic hepatitis C is usually diagnosed in a patient who was infected several years in the past. They usually are asymptomatic and see a doctor because somewhere along the line elevated ALT or AST activity was detected on blood tests taken for another reason. Often, blood tests are performed as part of a life insurance examination or to evaluate nonspecific symptoms such as fatigue, irritability, depression, or loss of appetite that is observed in individuals with chronic viral hepatitis. Some patients diagnosed by doctors will be similar to those in cases 3 and 4 that already have clinical signs and symptoms of chronic liver disease.

There are probably many more patients like the one presented in case 1; however, they are usually not diagnosed. If all patients who have a risk factor for hepatitis C virus infection, for example, anyone who ever received a blood transfusion prior to 1990, or anyone who ever used intravenous drugs, were tested for the virus, many more cases of chronic infection would be diagnosed. Many would probably be similar to the patient described in case 1; others like the patient described in case 2. Some authorities have, in fact, recommended that all individuals with risk factors for hepatitis C infection, for example, all recipients of blood transfusions prior to 1990, be tested.

Studies, and the experiences of doctors over the past several years, suggest that there are probably three "worlds" of individuals with chronic hepatitis C. One contains patients similar to those in described in case 1. The second world contains patients like those in case 2. The third contains those as in cases 3 and 4.

In one published study, sixty healthy blood donors infected with the hepatitis C virus were identified by blood screening. Liver biopsies were performed on all of them and only one had evidence of significant liver disease. These patients—most of whom will probably do well and never suffer from complications of liver disease—comprise the first "world."

On the other hand, a published study of over one hundred patients referred to a center that specializes in liver disease indicated that over 50 percent of patients already had cirrhosis and that many had hepatocellular carcinoma. These patients comprise the third "world" and are similar to those in cases 3 and 4. These are patients who are already very sick from chronic hepatitis C, most of whom will ultimately need liver transplantation to survive.

The second "world" of patients with chronic hepatitis C consists of people similar to the patient described in case 2. These are individuals with chronic infection, diagnosed by doctors, who do not yet have evidence of serious liver disease. *This "world" contains most of the patients who know that they have chronic hepatitis C and are monitored for it by doctors.* Most of these patients have liver biopsies that indicate ongoing inflammation of the liver, fibrosis (scarring), developing cirrhosis, or sometimes established cirrhosis without clinical symptoms or complications. Although there are no definitive numbers, most investigators estimate that about 25 percent of patients with chronic hepatitis C who are diagnosed by doctors will develop cirrhosis. Of this 25 percent who develop cirrhosis, some will develop liver failure and require liver transplantation and some will develop hepatocellular carcinoma. It is this second "world" of patients that treatment with interferon and other drugs will probably help the most.

A major challenge for doctors who treat patients with chronic hepatitis C is to determine which of the second "world" patients, such as the patient described in case 2, will enter the third "world" of patients with cirrhosis, advanced liver disease, or cancer. It is also not entirely clear if some of the first "world" patients, such as the patient described in case 1, will someday develop cirrhosis and complications after many years. Unfortunately, there are no absolute predictors of which will do relatively well and which will go on to develop cirrhosis and complications over time. However, a comprehensive evaluation can provide some useful predictive information.

The best test to obtain predictive data about a specific

patient with chronic hepatitis C infection (who does not already have clinically apparent complications of cirrhosis) is liver biopsy. Liver biopsy will establish the degree of inflammation, the degree of fibrosis (scarring), and the presence or absence of cirrhosis. Patients with significant inflammation or significant fibrosis are more likely to develop cirrhosis over time than those who do not have fibrosis or only minimal fibrosis. Patients who already have cirrhosis are at much greater risk for developing complications, liver failure, and hepatocellular carcinoma.

Viral genotype and concentration of hepatitis C virus RNA in the blood ("viral load") have been considered predictors of disease progression in chronic hepatitis C. Some investigators have shown that infection with hepatitis C virus genotypes 1a or 1b is correlated with a poorer prognosis than infection with non-type 1 genotypes. Although there are methodological and design limitations to all published studies that have addressed this issue, and not all studies agree, individuals infected with genotypes 1a or 1b *probably* have a higher chance of developing cirrhosis. This correlation is far from strict, however. Some patients infected with hepatitis C virus type 1 genotypes will not develop cirrhosis, and some with non-type 1 genotypes will have rapidly progressive liver disease.

The same holds true for "viral loads." Patients who have relatively high concentrations of viral RNA in the blood may be more likely to develop cirrhosis than those with lower "viral loads." But blood viral RNA concentrations can show considerable fluctuation in a given individual, and "viral load" is in no way a completely reliable predictor of who will or who will not develop cirrhosis. In general, patients infected with type 1 genotypes of the hepatitis C virus with high "viral loads" probably have a greater chance of developing cirrhosis than those infected with non-type 1 genotypes and lower "viral loads." There is extremely wide variability.

It is important to emphasize the effects of excessive alcohol consumption as a cofactor for liver damage in patients with chronic hepatitis C. Several studies and clinical observations suggest that alcohol is an independent risk factor for progression of liver disease and development of cirrhosis. Other studies have suggested that alcohol consumption accelerates the progression to cirrhosis in patients with chronic hepatitis C. In fact, the diagnosis of "cirrhosis caused by alcohol *and* hepatitis C" is heard more and more in medical wards these days. Perhaps the most famous person who suffered from this unfortunate "combination" was the late Mickey Mantle.

What is not clear about alcohol as a risk factor for the progression of liver disease in patients with hepatitis C is the *amount* of alcohol consumption that increases risk. Certainly, alcohol consumption of six or more drinks a day will increase the risk of liver disease, but probably at an even faster rate than in individuals who do not have chronic hepatitis C infection. The data, however, are less clear for lower amounts of alcohol consumption. Virtually all liver specialists will agree that no patient with chronic hepatitis C should have more than two alcoholic drinks a day. Many experts in this field would even argue that patients with chronic hepatitis C should consume *no* alcohol. My personal feeling at this time, given the lack of data from well-controlled, forward-looking studies, is that patients with chronic hepatitis C should limit their alcohol intake to no more than a few drinks a few times per week. A couple of glasses of wine with an *occasional* nice dinner, a beer at a ball game, or an *occasional* cocktail at a party will probably not be detrimental to the person with chronic hepatitis C. However, this level of drinking may become problematic if it occurs on a daily basis. Patients with chronic hepatitis C certainly should not exceed two drinks per day and should probably keep their alcohol intake *well below* this amount.

The most important things to remember about the course of chronic hepatitis C virus infection are:

1. Chronic hepatitis C virus infection is frequently "silent" as the patient has no or only nonspecific symptoms.
2. The course of chronic hepatitis C virus infection can vary significantly. Some individuals may develop cirrhosis after only a few years of infection. Some individuals may develop cirrhosis after many years. Other infected individuals will never develop significant liver disease or complications.
3. It is extremely difficult to predict the rate or progression of liver disease in an individual with chronic hepatitis C. Liver biopsy is the best source of predictive information. Genotype and viral load may provide limited information.
4. Liver disease progresses more rapidly in patients with chronic hepatitis C who consume too much alcohol, but what constitutes a "safe" lower limit is not known at present.

Transmission

It is estimated that 4 million people in the U.S. are infected with the hepatitis C virus. Worldwide estimates range from 100 million to 150 million people. Hepatitis C virus infection occurs in virtually all regions of the world. In some areas, one prominent example being Egypt, the prevalence of infection is significantly higher than in other areas.

Hepatitis C virus is transmitted primarily by blood and blood products. There are several other documented modes of transmission. The major risk factors are listed in Table 4.6.

Because a test for detection of antibodies against the hepatitis C virus was first used to screen the blood supply in 1990, and an even more sensitive test was used in 1992, the risk of infection via a blood transfusion has become increasingly small. It

Table 4.6. *Risk factors for hepatitis C virus infection.*

Blood transfusions before 1990 or 1992[1] (in developed countries)
Intravenous drug use
Tattoos
Body piercing
Sexual and household contacts of infected individuals[2]
Sexually promiscuous individuals[2]
Transmission from infected mother to newborn baby[2]
Health care workers exposed to blood[2]
Infected health care workers to patients (rare)
Hemodialysis
Intranasal cocaine use[3]
Ear piercing in men[3]

---

[1] Blood supply screening began in 1990 and was improved by use of better tests in 1992.

[2] These risk factors are real but less than those for the hepatitis B virus (see text).

[3] It is unclear if these are actually modes of transmission or factors associated with other lifestyle activities that may increase transmission (for example, intranasal cocaine abusers may also be more likely to have used intravenous drugs at some prior time).

has been estimated that, between 1991 and 1993, the chance of receiving a unit of blood contaminated with the hepatitis C virus was greater than 1 in 100,000. However, patients who received blood transfusions before 1990, *even in the remote past,* are at risk *now* for having hepatitis C. One important thing to remember about hepatitis C is that it is a chronic, often slowly progressive disease. Even patients who are now elderly and had blood transfusions when they were babies may still carry the hepatitis C virus in their bodies.

Intravenous drug use remains a very important mode of transmission for the hepatitis C virus. Inner-city intravenous drug users are at very high risk and infection rates may well approach 90 percent in active, recurrent users. Again, as with blood transfusion, it is critical to realize that intravenous drug use even once in the remote past presents a definite risk for hepatitis C virus infection. A very typical history is that of an upper-class, middle-aged man or woman, now an upstanding member of the community with a very important job, who sees a doctor because of an abnormally elevated ALT activity on blood tests for life insurance. Upon questioning, the doctor learns that this individual used intravenous drugs "a couple of times in college in the sixties when everyone was using them." For thirty or more years, the patient was healthy and living a clean life. Little did that person know that all along the hepatitis C virus was in his or her body.

One study has demonstrated that intranasal cocaine use is a risk factor for hepatitis C infection. Some investigators have hypothesized that sharing straws can transmit the virus as a small amount of bleeding can occur inside the nose while snorting cocaine. This mode of transmission has not been clearly proven, and it is possible that intranasal cocaine use may be a risk factor for hepatitis C virus infection only because such individuals are more likely to use, or to have used, intravenous drugs. Nonetheless, intranasal cocaine use should be considered a possible mode of transmission for the hepatitis C virus.

There are several other modes of transmission and risk factors for infection with the hepatitis C virus. As the virus is transmitted by blood, other modes of exposure can transmit it. Hepatitis C virus can be spread by tattooing and body piercing if sterile techniques are not practiced. One study has claimed that men, but not women, with pierced ears are at increased risk for hepatitis C virus infection. Whether men are more likely to have piercing performed under nonsterile conditions, or whether ear piercing in men is associated with other high-risk behaviors (for example, intravenous drug use may be more common in men with pierced ears), is not clear. Nonetheless, tattooing and piercing present potential modes of transmission for the hepatitis C virus.

The hepatitis C virus is also spread in settings where individuals are exposed to blood on a regular basis. Health care and hospital workers are at increased risk for infection. Transmission by needle sticks have been documented. Transmission by medical instruments, for example, colonoscopes, has also been reported. Rare cases of transmission of hepatitis C virus from surgeons to patients have also occurred. The transmission risks of hepatitis C virus by these modes are probably much less than for the hepatitis B virus.

Many individuals with chronic hepatitis C, and the household members and sexual contacts who interact with these individuals, have major concerns about transmission. Household members appear to be at a slightly increased risk for contracting hepatitis C. Hidden modes of blood transmission can occur among household members with possible instruments of transmission including shared razors, toothbrushes, baby bottles, and children's toys. Transmission of hepatitis C probably does not occur by touching, holding hands, kissing, or hugging.

The data regarding sexual transmission suggest that individuals with multiple sex partners are at increased risk for hepatitis C virus, but that individuals in long-term monogamous sexual relationships with an infected partner are at low risk. The rate of sexual transmission of the hepatitis C virus appears to be much lower than that for the hepatitis B virus. The prevalence of chronic hepatitis C virus infection is significantly higher in homosexual men, patients in sexually transmitted disease clinics, and female professional sex workers compared to the general population. This suggests that sexual transmission of the virus is a probable route, although it is not entirely clear if the risk of infection is higher in these groups because of other concurrent lifestyle factors (for example, past or current intravenous drug use). Studies of partners of infected individuals in long-term, monogamous sexual relationships suggest that the rate of transmission of hepatitis C virus to a noninfected partner is rather low. Some studies suggest that the sexual partner is at no greater risk for infection than other household members (i.e., the young son of an infected father has the same risk of getting infected as the wife). Based on these observations, the U.S. Centers for Disease Control and Prevention currently recommend that sexually promiscuous individuals should use condoms to prevent contracting or spreading hepatitis C virus (*and* HIV, hepatitis B virus, *Chlamydia,* gonorrhea, syphilis, etc.). Condoms are not considered essential but are an option for monogamous couples in which one partner is infected with the hepatitis C virus and who do not plan on changing their current sexual habits.

Women with chronic hepatitis C virus infection of childbearing potential are always concerned about the risks of transmitting the virus to their newborn babies. Fortunately, the risk of transmission from mother to infant is much lower than that for the hepatitis B virus. Several studies have shown rates of infection of the hepatitis C virus from infected mothers to their new-borns to be less than 10 percent. Some studies report rates as low at 1 percent or 2 percent. Pregnant women with hepatitis C virus infection should be aware that there is a small but real risk of transmitting the virus to their babies.

Of all patients who present to doctors and in whom chronic hepatitis C infection is diagnosed, as many as one-third report no known risk factor. Studies in the U.S. have shown that, upon detailed questioning, some individuals will ultimately admit to past intravenous drug use. However, some have not used drugs. A possible mode of transmission is having been treated with un-sterile medical equipment in the past. This is probably a mode of transmission in underdeveloped countries where needles for vaccination and drawing blood are frequently reused. Other hidden past exposures to blood and blood products are also possible in virtually anyone.

Diagnosis

The diagnosis of chronic hepatitis C is suspected in several types of patients:

- Individuals with risk factors (see Table 4.6)
- Individuals with elevated ALT and/or AST activities on blood tests
- Individuals with signs and symptoms of liver disease
- Individuals with unexplained nonspecific symptoms
- Individuals with a diagnosis of alcoholic liver disease

One group are patients with no evidence of illness but who have risk factors for chronic hepatitis C virus infection such as intravenous drug use, blood transfusions prior to 1992 (when a very good screening test was used on the blood sup-ply), or other risks outlined in Table 4.6. *Chronic hepatitis C virus infection should even be suspected in individuals with risk factors who are asymptomatic and/or have normal ALT and AST activities on blood testing.* In addition, chronic hepatitis C should be considered a possible diagnosis in any individual who has elevated ALT and/or AST activities, even if the elevations are only minimal and the patient has no obvious risk factors. Finally, chronic hepatitis C virus infection should be suspected in all individuals with signs and symptoms of liver disease, again, even if there are no identifiable risk factors and if the ALT and/or AST activities are normal. Some may have unexplained nonspecific complaints such as fatigue or mild depression. As hepatitis C virus infection is often found concurrently in individuals with alcoholic liver disease, patients with a diagnosis of alcoholic liver disease should also be tested for antibodies against the hepatitis C virus.

Several blood tests are now available for the diagnosis of infection with the hepatitis C virus (Table 4.7). Each of these tests has its advantages and disadvantages. Some of these tests should be used only in special circumstances.

Table 4.7. *Blood tests for hepatitis C virus infection*

Antibody tests	Enzyme-linked immunosorbent assay (ELISA)
	Recombinant immunoblot (RIBA)
RNA tests	Branched chain DNA (bDNA)
	Reverse transcription-polymerase chain reaction (RT-PCR)

The first test that was available in the diagnosis of hepatitis C virus infection was the enzyme-linked immunosorbent assay or ELISA. Since it first became available in 1990, the ELISA has been repeatedly improved. ELISA detects the presence of antibodies against proteins of the hepatitis C virus. The actual test now contains several viral proteins coated on a plastic dish. The patient's blood is incubated in the dish, the dish is then washed, and a second antibody that recognizes human antibodies is then added. The second antibody is attached to an enzyme that will change the color of an indicator that is added next. If the patient has antibodies against hepatitis C virus proteins, they will stick to the viral proteins coated on the dish. The stuck antibodies will then be recognized by the second antibodies, which will change the color of the added indicator. If the color changes, the patient has antibodies against the hepatitis C virus. The ELISA will be negative in *acute* hepatitis C as it takes six weeks or longer for an infected person to develop antibodies.

Currently available ELISAs are about 95 to 99 percent sensitive for the diagnosis of chronic hepatitis C. This means that of all patients with chronic hepatitis C, 95 to 99 percent will have positive ELISA tests. ELISA is the first test that most doctors will use in the diagnosis of chronic hepatitis C. ELISA is also the test used currently to screen the blood supply, and donated blood that tests positive in this assay is discarded. *It should be assumed that an individual with a positive ELISA test has chronic hepatitis C until proven otherwise.*

In rare cases, the ELISA test for antibodies against the hepatitis C virus will be "false positive." False positive means that the test will be positive even though the patient does not have hepatitis C. This occurs if antibodies indiscriminately stick to the plastic dish or any protein. This is a rare occurrence and should be suspected in individuals who have normal ALT on blood testing *and* no risk factors. In these individuals with a positive hepatitis C ELISA test, a confirmatory test should be performed. A false positive test should also be suspected in individuals with rare diseases that cause elevations in immunoglobulins in the blood. One disease in which immunoglobulins may be elevated, and which is sometimes confused clinically with the diagnosis of hepatitis C, is autoimmune hepatitis. In individuals with a positive hepatitis C ELISA and elevated blood immunoglobulins, a confirmatory test should also be performed.

A test that adds specificity to the detection of antibodies against the hepatitis C virus is the recombinant immunoblot assay or RIBA. In this test, several proteins of the hepatitis C virus are coated onto a plastic strip. A "control" or irrelevant protein is added to the same strip. The strip is then incubated with the patient's blood and processed similar to the ELISA. However, with the RIBA you can determine the exact proteins recognized by the antibodies. If the patient has antibodies that react with two viral proteins and not the control protein, it is positive. If the patient's blood contains antibodies that react with the control protein only, it is negative. If it contains antibodies that react with only one viral protein, or more than one viral protein and the control protein, it is indeterminate. RIBA is not used often anymore given the advent of RNA tests, which can test directly for the presence of the virus. Like the ELISA, the RIBA will also be negative in acute hepatitis C infection.

The commercial availability of tests to detect hepatitis C virus RNA in blood has improved the diagnosis of hepatitis C virus infection. These tests are for a viral component itself and not for antibodies. The most sensitive test is reverse transcription-polymerase chain reaction or RT-PCR, commonly called PCR. In this test, RNA is extracted from the blood and copied to DNA by an enzyme known as reverse transcriptase. A biochemical reaction known as the polymerase chain reaction (PCR) is then used to amplify the viral DNA copy so that it can be detected by routine chemical methods. The other test for hepatitis C viral RNA in the blood is branched chain DNA, commonly called bDNA. In this test, a fraction of the blood is incubated with a synthetic DNA molecule that binds to hepatitis C viral RNA. If viral RNA is present, it is captured in a tiny dish and then detected by a chemical reaction involving a second synthetic DNA molecule.

The main advantage of PCR is that it is more sensitive than bDNA. Another advantage is that it can be modified to determine the genotype of the infecting hepatitis C virus (usually for an extra charge). The major disadvantage of PCR is that it is more expensive and requires greater expertise to perform. Both PCR and bDNA can be modified to estimate "viral load" which is the concentration of viral RNA in the blood. The trend today is to use PCR to detect hepatitis C viral RNA in blood, with the caveat that it should be performed in a reliable clinical laboratory.

Who should have tests for hepatitis C virus RNA? The following criteria should be considered:

- Positive ELISA but normal ALT on blood testing and no risk factor
- Positive ELISA but elevated blood globulins
- Negative ELISA, strong clinical suspicion of chronic hepatitis C
- Suspected acute hepatitis C
- Six months after stopping treatment to see if virus is cleared
- Prior to treatment and following response to treatment

RNA tests are *not* screening tests. One role of RNA tests is to confirm or refute the results of an antibody test. In these instances, the PCR test is probably a better choice than the bDNA assay because it is more sensitive. If an antibody test is negative and the clinical suspicion of chronic hepatitis C is low (no risk factor and normal ALT and AST; elevated ALT and AST but obvious other diagnosis), the patient probably does not have chronic hepatitis C. If the doctor has a strong clinical suspicion of hepatitis C despite a negative antibody test, however, then a PCR test should be performed because about 1 to 5 percent of patients infected with hepatitis C virus will have negative antibody tests. PCR testing is also a good idea to confirm the diagnosis of chronic hepatitis C in patients in whom an antibody test may be false positive, such as those with high concentrations of blood immunoglobulins. An RNA test should probably be performed also in a patient with a positive antibody test but no risk factor for hepatitis C virus infection and normal serum ALT activity. An RNA test must also be performed to diagnose acute hepatitis C as the antibody tests will be negative in acute cases.

The other major role of hepatitis C virus RNA tests is for tracking response to treatment. PCR, or possibly bDNA, should probably be performed prior to treatment. Some authorities then recommend a repeat test after three months of treatment to determine if the patient has responded. RNA tests, preferably PCR because of its increased sensitivity, should also be performed immediately after treatment, six months after treatment is discontinued, and periodically thereafter to determine if the patient has "cleared" the virus and if this response persists.

After infection with the hepatitis C virus has been established by antibody or RNA testing, a liver biopsy is usually indicated in the diagnosis of a patient with chronic hepatitis C. The major reasons for performing a liver biopsy are outlined above and in chapter 2. A liver biopsy may also prove useful in the evaluation of patients with two concurrent diseases, for example, someone who abuses alcohol and is infected with hepatitis C virus.

Treatment

The demonstration that alpha-interferons are effective in the treatment of patients with chronic hepatitis C has radically changed the practice of hepatology. It is probably for this reason alone that more gastroenterologists today also consider themselves "hepatologists" compared to just a few years ago. It also marked the first time that any proven treatment could be offered to patients with chronic viral hepatitis.

Almost all patients with chronic hepatitis C should be considered for treatment. *If the diagnosis of chronic hepatitis C is made by a primary doctor who is not familiar with treatment, the patient should be referred to a specialist who is.* Not all patients are necessarily candidates for treatment, but most should at least be evaluated by a specialist experienced with treatment of hepatitis C who can make this determination. Possible exceptions to this rule include patients with more pressing concurrent illnesses, for example, heart disease or cancer, elderly patients, and patients with advanced cirrhosis who should be referred for evaluation for liver transplantation if they are eligible.

At present, the FDA has approved three different recombinant alpha interferons to treat patients with chronic hepatitis C (Table 4.8). Alpha interferons have a multitude of effects on the body including activation of general antiviral responses and stimulation of the immune system to seek out and kill virus-infected cells. Recently, the FDA has also approved the combination of interferon alpha-2b and ribavirin for patients with chronic hepatitis C (Table 4.8). Ribavirin is a synthetic compound that has activity against a few different viruses. In the U.S., it was first approved in aerosol form for treatment of a type of respiratory virus infection in children. In several studies,

Table 4.8. *Drugs approved for treating chronic hepatitis C.**

Generic name	Trade name	Manufacturer
interferon alpha-2b	Intron-A	Schering-Plough
interferon alpha-2a	Roferon	Hoffman La Roche
interferon alfacon-1	Infergen	Amgen
interferon alpha-2b/ ribavirin combination	Rebetron	Schering-Plough

*Drugs are listed in the order they were approved for this indication by the FDA.

oral ribavirin was examined as a single agent for the treatment of adults with chronic hepatitis C but proved only partially effective. However, combination therapy with interferon alpha-2b and ribavirin was subsequently shown in several studies to be more effective than interferon alpha-2b alone in the treatment of adults with chronic hepatitis C.

Alpha interferons come either as powders that must be mixed with sterile water before use, or, more often, as premixed solutions. Both powder and premixed solutions are stable if stored in the refrigerator. Interferon alpha is administered by subcutaneous (under the skin) or intramuscular (into the muscle) injections. Most patients administer the injections to themselves with small syringes and needles similar to those used by diabetics to inject insulin. Some may use an "injection pen" supplied with the drug. Most people choose to inject the interferon into the thigh; however, other areas such as the abdomen can also be injected. Patients should make every effort to obtain brief training from a doctor or nurse before starting injections by themselves.

Ribavirin for chronic hepatitis C comes as 200 mg (0.2 g) capsules. The capsules are stable at room temperature. The drug is taken twice a day—in the morning and at night. The recommended dose is two capsules in the morning and three in the evening (1 g total) for individuals who weigh less than 165 lb. (75 kg) and three tablets in the morning and three in the evening (1.2 g) for individuals who weigh 165 lb. (75 kg) or more.

The approval of three different interferon alphas in the U.S. for treatment of chronic hepatitis C, and the more recent approval of interferon alpha-2b plus ribavirin, has made the discussion of treatment somewhat complicated. There is no absolute right or wrong choice as to which interferon preparation to use, or if interferon alpha-2b plus ribavirin should be used for the first course of treatment. Some doctors may use interferon alpha-2b plus ribavirin as the first line of treatment while others may reserve combination treatment for the second time around. *The current trend, which will probably be more prevalent in the next couple of years, is to use combination therapy with ribavirin as first-line therapy.*

There are a few things to consider before embarking on a further discussion about the treatment of chronic hepatitis C:

1. Studies published so far have shown better response rates with interferon alpha-2b plus ribavirin than with interferon alpha-2b alone (and by extrapolation, although not yet tested head-to-head, other forms of interferon alpha). *The trend among most liver specialists is probably to use combination therapy when appropriate for a given patient.*

2. Despite claims to the contrary by manufacturers, all three approved preparations of interferon alpha are probably similar. They all work by the same mechanism of action, and no randomized, controlled clinical trial has yet shown any single one to be better or worse.

3. Treatment with interferon alpha is associated with side effects and treatment with interferon alpha-2b plus ribavirin is associated with additional side effects.
4. Most patients relapse after treatment with an interferon. Most, but fewer than with an interferon alone, also relapse after treatment with interferon alpha-2b plus ribavirin.
5. Despite the fact that most patients relapse after treatment, it is not possible to predict if a single patient will have a long-term response. Therefore, treatment should probably be offered to all patients who are eligible.
6. There may be some benefit to treatment even in individuals who do not have long-term responses.

Before proceeding further, I should also define some jargon that has caught on in the field of treating chronic hepatitis C. Although these terms are not all scientifically accurate or precise, they are used by most liver specialists and patients, so I will use them too (although I think some of them are silly). The best measure of response to treatment today is the loss of hepatitis C virus RNA from the blood when measured by PCR testing. In older studies conducted before routine RNA testing was readily available, response to treatment was assessed by measuring blood ALT activities. Some of the terms used to describe treatment responses in patients with chronic hepatitis C are defined in Table 4.9.

Which patients with chronic hepatitis C should be treated (Table 4.10)? To be eligible for treatment, patients should have diagnosis of chronic (more than six months) hepatitis C. This is usually the case in individuals with hepatitis C at the time of diagnosis. Prior to starting treatment, patients with chronic hepatitis C should have a liver biopsy to confirm diagnosis and determine the severity of disease (I should add that a few doctors disagree with this). Patients who have clinical complications

Table 4.9. *Terms (not always precise) used in describing responses to treatment in patients with chronic hepatitis C.* *

Term	Definition
"Responder"	A patient who has undetectable virus in blood during treatment.
"Non-responder"	A patient who still has detectable virus RNA in blood during treatment.
"Relapser"	A patient who "responded" to treatment and then had detectable serum virus RNA after treatment was discontinued.
"Treatment failure"	"Non-responder" *or* "relapser."
"Sustained responder"	A patient with undetectable blood virus RNA six months or longer after stopping treatment.
"Partial responder"	A patient whose blood virus concentration or ALT activity decreases during treatment but in whom virus is still detectable.
"Breakthrough"	This term is used if a patient has an initial response to treatment and then again develops detectable blood virus RNA during treatment.

*The terms are best used to define detectable hepatitis C virus RNA in blood but are also sometimes used in regard to ALT activity.

of cirrhosis such as ascites, hepatic encephalopathy, and/or bleeding esophageal varices should probably not be treated outside of approved research studies. Patients with evidence of compromised liver function on blood tests, such as a low albumin concentration, significantly elevated bilirubin concentration, or prolonged prothrombin time more than three seconds greater than normal, also should probably not be treated except in approved studies. Patients with significantly low platelet counts, low white blood counts, and significant anemia also should not receive interferon. The exact cutoff values for exclusion are not agreed upon by all doctors, however. Individuals with even milder anemia may not be able to receive ribavirin. Patients with hypothyroidism, hyperthyroidism, or poorly controlled diabetes should also not be treated until these conditions are medically controlled. Treatment may also not be indicated for patients with depression or other psychiatric problems. Patients with heart disease may not be good candidates either, especially for treatment with ribavirin that can rapidly cause anemia leading to a heart attack for someone who is at risk. Patients with other serious disorders such as cancer, or other debilitating diseases, should also defer treatment.

Patients with chronic hepatitis C who have never been treated previously are referred to in the (often silly) jargon used by liver specialists as "naive." So-called naive patients being treated for the first time should receive a dose of interferon alpha equivalent to 3 million units *three times a week*. For interferon alpha-2a and interferon alpha-2b, the dose is prescribed as 3 million units three times a week. For interferon alfacon-1, the drug is prescribed on a mass basis of 9 mcg, which is roughly equivalent to 3 million units, three times a week. For interferon alpha-2b plus ribavirin, the interferon alpha-2b is given at a dose of 3 million units three times a week and the ribavirin is taken *orally* twice a day, *every day*, at a total dose of 1.0 g or

Table 4.10. *Criteria to consider patients with chronic hepatitis C for treatment with interferon or interferon alpha-2b plus ribavirin.*

Patients should have:

Chronic hepatitis C (greater than six months of infection) with a consistent liver biopsy

No ascites, encephalopathy, and/or bleeding esophageal varices

Normal, stable blood albumin concentration

Normal or near normal blood bilirubin concentration

Prothrombin time no more than three seconds greater than a normal control

Treatment may not be suitable for patients with:

Significantly low platelet count, low white blood count, or moderate to severe anemia

Hypothyroidism

Hyperthyroidism

Diabetes mellitus

Systemic medical diseases

Heart disease (especially important if considering ribavirin)

Cancer

Depression or other psychiatric conditions

AIDS (but okay if HIV infection without severe immune system dysfunction)

1.2 g a day depending upon the patient's weight. At the present time, preparations of interferon alpha-2a and interferon alpha-2b made as slow-release mixtures with polyethylene glycol (so-called pegylated interferon) are being tested in patients with chronic hepatitis C. These preparations have not yet been approved in the U.S. If approved, they will likely require less frequent injections when used either with or without ribavirin. They may also lead to better response rates as blood interferon levels will fluctuate less.

How do patients with chronic hepatitis C being treated for the first time respond? About two-thirds are "responders" to treatment meaning that blood viral RNA will not be detectable and blood ALT activity will probably also return to normal. Roughly a third of patients will be "non-responders" in whom viral RNA will persist in the blood during treatment. Some of the *initial* "responders" will experience "breakthrough" during treatment and viral RNA will be detected in the blood later in the course of therapy. The initial response rates are roughly similar with an interferon alpha alone or with interferon alpha-2b plus ribavirin.

Although there are no absolute rules, most liver specialists will check a hepatitis C virus RNA concentration in the blood before treatment and after three months of treatment. If viral RNA is still detectable at three months, the patient is considered a "non-responder." In such patients, it may be reasonable to consider an alternative to the current therapy, for example, adding ribavirin if interferon alpha alone is being used.

Again, there are no strict rules, and some doctors may continue treatment for another three months or longer even if there is no response. If patients respond at three months by having undetectable blood hepatitis C virus RNA, the current treatment should be continued. If the patient continues to tolerate treatment without subsequent viral RNA detected in the blood during treatment, therapy should probably be continued for *at least* twenty-four weeks. The duration of treatment for responders is not universally agreed upon; some doctors will continue treatment for a total of twenty-four weeks, and others as long as two years.

At the completion of treatment, blood tests should be performed to measure viral RNA by PCR. ALT activity should also be checked. Patients without detectable viral RNA by PCR testing at the completion of treatment are called "end-of-treatment responders." In end-of-treatment responders, PCR testing for viral RNA should be performed again six months after stopping therapy. Patients who do not have detectable serum viral RNA six months after finishing treatment are called "sustained responders" or "long-term responders." Sustained responders may "relapse" and again have detectable blood viral RNA at a later time, however. Therefore, ALT activities and RNA concentrations should probably be checked periodically, perhaps every six to twelve months after treatment is stopped.

How many patients will be "sustained responders" and have no detectable serum hepatitis C virus RNA in the blood six months or longer after treatment? In patients treated with an interferon alone for twenty-four weeks, less than 20 percent will be "sustained responders." Treatment for forty-eight weeks improves the response rate to around 20 percent. In patients treated with interferon alpha-2b plus ribavirin for twenty-four weeks, the six-month sustained response rate approaches 40 percent in the few studies published thus far. It may be slightly higher with forty-eight weeks of combination treatment.

There are several predictors to determine which patients with chronic hepatitis C are more likely to respond to treatment. In general, the following are correlated with a *lower* probability of responding: age greater than forty-five years, duration of infection longer than five years, the presence of fibrosis or cirrhosis on liver biopsy, higher blood hepatitis C virus RNA concentrations, and infection with genotypes 1a or 1b. Despite these facts, it is not possible to apply these predictors to an individual patient to calculate his or her exact chance of responding to treatment. A doctor may be able to better guess ahead of time who is more or less likely to respond but cannot make these predictions with certainty.

One of the big issues in the treatment of patients with chronic hepatitis C is what to offer patients who are "nonresponders" or "relapsers." The current options are basically limited to:

1. Retreatment with interferon alpha-2b plus ribavirin for patients who received an interferon alone for their first course of treatment.
2. Retreatment with an alpha-interferon, at a higher dose and/or for a longer duration.
3. Enrollment in approved clinical studies.

The results of at least one large, prospective, randomized study has shown that the combination of interferon plus ribavirin improves the response rate of "relapsers" previously treated with an alpha-interferon alone. In a study of 345 patients, 45.7 percent of "relapsers" who received interferon alpha-2b plus ribavirin had undetectable blood hepatitis C virus RNA six months after stopping therapy as compared to 4.7 percent who received only interferon alpha-2b. For patients with chronic hepatitis C who "relapse" after treatment with an interferon alone, retreatment with the combination of interferon alpha-2b plus ribavirin is the best option available at this time. In fact, treatment of "relapsers" was the first indication for which combination therapy was approved by the FDA.

Reliable data on retreatment of "non-responders" to interferon alpha alone are not presently available, but many liver specialists would probably offer treatment with the interferon alpha-2b plus ribavirin combination to their non-responders. Non-responders do, however, have lower sustained response rates to retreatment than relapsers. Patients who initially respond and experience a breakthrough with detectable serum viral RNA during treatment should probably be approached the same as non-responders.

Retreatment with an interferon alpha alone, perhaps at a higher dose and/or for longer duration, may also prove useful in the retreatment of non-responders and relapsers. If patients were previously treated for only twenty-four weeks, treatment for forty-eight weeks or longer may improve the chance of being a sustained responder the second time around. A few studies have indicated that response rates to a second course of treatment with interferon will be higher if the dose of interferon alfacon-1 is increased to 15 mcg three times per week or if the dose of interferon alpha-2b is increased to 5 million units three times a week. Many studies have looked at numerous variations in the doses of interferons for chronic hepatitis C. In general, it can really only be stated that longer duration and higher dose retreatment with an alpha interferon may improve the long-term response rate. Relapsers are more likely to have a sustained response than non-responders. On the downside, higher doses and long-term treatment are associated with increased side effects.

What about patients with chronic hepatitis C who "fail" a second course of therapy? At the present time, no specific recommendations can be made. If they did not receive ribavirin as part of the first two treatment courses, they should probably receive treatment with interferon alpha-2b plus ribavirin. If they have already received interferon plus ribavirin, one possibility is to consider the patient for enrollment in approved clinical trials. Some of these trials are examining higher doses of interferon alpha combined with ribavirin, and others are examining experimental drugs. Another possibility is observation until new and more promising drugs become available. The choice between these options depends upon the particular patient and his or her doctor.

There are numerous side effects associated with the preparations of interferon alpha. For this reason, careful monitoring is necessary during treatment.

Because low blood counts are one potential side effect, patients should have their blood drawn and complete blood counts and platelet counts checked at intervals of one, two, and four weeks after treatment is started and once a month thereafter. Blood ALT activity, bilirubin concentration, and albumin concentration should also be checked periodically during therapy. Patients should probably be seen by their doctors or nurses at least once a month during treatment and instructed to contact their doctor if they experience side effects.

Common and potentially serious side effects of interferon alpha at doses generally used to treat patients with chronic hepatitis C are low neutrophil counts and low platelet counts. Neutrophils, also called granulocytes, are a particular type of white blood cell important in fighting bacterial infections. Platelets are involved in blood clotting and may also be low in individuals with cirrhosis. As mentioned above, patients should have their blood counts monitored during treatment with interferon alpha. If the neutrophil count falls below 750 cells per cubic millimeter of blood or the platelet count falls below 50,000 cells per cubic millimeter of blood, the daily dose can be cut in half until baseline values rise above these levels. If the neutrophil count falls below 500 cells per cubic millimeter of blood or the platelet count below 30,000 cells per cubic millimeter of blood, interferon alpha therapy should probably be discontinued. Resumption of treatment can be considered when blood counts return to their baseline values.

There are *many* other side effects of interferon alpha therapy besides low blood counts. The most common is the development of flu-like symptoms. These can be quite severe and include fever, cold sweats, shaking chills, muscle aches and pains, and joint aches and pains. Flu-like symptoms are usually worse at the start of treatment and less common later in the course of therapy. To help tolerate mild to moderate flu-like symptoms, I generally recommend that patients inject the interferon about an hour before going to sleep and take acetaminophen right before injecting the interferon. The acetaminophen will provide some relief from symptoms and, if taken at bedtime, possibly help the patient to sleep through the night. Flu-like symptoms rarely require stopping treatment but on occasion they are so intolerable that there is no other option.

Interferon alpha treatment can aggravate diabetes mellitus and thyroid disorders. Patients with diabetes mellitus who are treated with interferon alpha should carefully monitor their blood sugars. Patients with thyroid disease, and 5possibly all treated patients, should have blood tests of thyroid function checked periodically during treatment. Significant abnormalities in blood sugar or thyroid tests may necessitate stopping treatment.

Nervous system and psychiatric problems—some severe— have been reported in individuals receiving alpha interferons. Tingling in the extremities is the most common nervous system side effect. Depression, irritability, confusion, nervousness, impaired concentration, anxiety, and insomnia have all occurred in individuals taking interferon alpha and perhaps more commonly in studies in which interferon alpha-2b was combined with ribavirin. Sometimes, these psychiatric problems are so severe that treatment must be stopped. Of note, severe depression has occurred in individuals taking interferon and suicides have been reported. Patients with *serious* preexisting depression or other psychiatric disorders probably should not be treated with interferon alpha. If significant depression develops during treatment, the drug(s) should be discontinued immediately and the patient closely followed and referred to a psychiatrist as necessary. In addition, patients with less significant psychiatric disorders, or with depression which is well controlled, should also probably be evaluated by a psychiatrist before starting treatment.

Virtually every complaint has been reported by patients receiving interferon alpha. Some of the more frequent side effects which are usually not severe include fever, rashes, headache, muscle aches, fatigue, back pain, dry mouth, nausea, diarrhea, and inflammation at the injection site. All are usually mild to moderate and do not require stopping treatment. Rare patients have had what appear to be allergic reactions to interferon alpha; the drug must be discontinued if these occur. Despite numerous side effects, interferon alpha therapy is rather safe if patients are monitored closely and most complete the course of therapy without incident.

There are additional side effects if ribavirin is added to interferon alpha, and in general about twice as many patients have to discontinue treatment. The major side effect of ribavirin is the rapid development of *hemolytic anemia*—sudden drop in the hemoglobin or hematocrit that results due to rupture of red blood cells. For this reason, the patient's blood count must be monitored one, two, and four weeks after starting therapy and at least monthly thereafter. If hemoglobin concentration drops to below 10 mg per deciliter during treatment, the ribavirin dose should be cut in half until it returns to normal. If the hemoglobin concentration drops to below 8.5 mg per deciliter, ribavirin treatment should be discontinued. Because sudden onset anemia can be very dangerous in individuals with heart disease, patients known to have significant heart disease should not receive ribavirin. Patients at risk for heart disease should be given a stress test prior to treatment.

The major goals of treatment for patients with chronic hepatitis C are to eradicate the virus from the body and slow progression of liver disease. It should now be obvious that eradication of the viral infection is achieved only in a minority of patients. Furthermore, most data available from published studies are available only for six months after treatment and "sustained response" rates are likely to be even lower with longer term follow-up. Another treatment goal is to slow or halt the progression of liver disease. Even if the virus is not eradicated from the body, improvements in liver inflammation and fibrosis are often obtained. Although long-term follow-up is not available, in some cases partially successful treatment may slow or halt the progression to cirrhosis in a given patient's lifetime. Some studies have also suggested that treatment of patients with cirrhosis caused by hepatitis C have a lower incidence for development of hepatocellular carcinoma after several years of follow-up.

Treatment of chronic hepatitis C is a rapidly evolving and changing field of medicine. Many clinical studies are still in progress to optimize treatment and develop options for retreatment of non-responders and relapsers. Many pharmaceutical companies are working on novel drugs to attack the hepatitis C virus. Once they have been approved, these drugs will add greater specificity to treatment and either complement, or be used in place of, the currently available interferon alpha-based therapies. It is unlikely that these "drugs of the future" will be available soon. The important information worth noting about the treatment of chronic hepatitis C is:

1. Treatment of patients with chronic hepatitis C with interferon alpha or interferon plus ribavirin is not yet an exact science. Different doctors recommend different durations of

treatment with different preparations of alpha interferon. There is no single agreed-upon approach. A particular doctor's judgment and biases, and sometimes the patient's wishes, are important factors in determining the exact treatment plan.

2. One important question for treatment of first-time patients is whether to use an alpha interferon alone or the combination of interferon alpha-2b plus ribavirin. *The current and growing trend is to use interferon alpha-2b with ribavirin whenever appropriate.* Combination treatment gives better sustained response rates but is associated with a greater frequency of side effects.

3. Patients who are non-responders or relapse after a first course of treatment should be considered for a second treatment. At the present time, the best option is "retreatment" with the combination of interferon alpha-2b plus ribavirin for those previously treated with interferon alone. Another option is retreatment with an interferon alpha at a higher dose and for longer duration.

4. It is not yet clear what to do with patients who do not respond, or relapse, after more than one course of treatment. These patients should probably be considered for enrollment in approved clinical studies. Observation without treatment is also an option.

5. Although a "virological cure" (eradication of the virus from the body) is a major goal of therapy, treatment may be associated with other benefits such as a decrease in the chance of developing cirrhosis or hepatocellular carcinoma.

6. *Patients who do not respond to presently available treatments should remain optimistic.* Chronic hepatitis C is usually a slowly progressive disease and new drugs will likely be available in the next few years.

Medical follow-up and cancer screening

Patients with chronic hepatitis C should have consistent medical follow-up whether or not they are candidates for drug treatment. Even individuals without symptoms, normal blood ALT and AST activities, and minimal inflammation on liver biopsies should see their doctors periodically. On the whole, such individuals will probably do extremely well in the long term; however, it is clear that an individual patient without any apparent liver disease at one point in time may develop a more aggressive disease later. Therefore, periodic physical examinations and laboratory tests are reasonable recommendations. If a patient has chronic hepatitis C over many years without significant clinical change, they should probably see a doctor about once a year. A physical examination should be performed to confirm there are no signs of cirrhosis. Blood tests should be checked for evidence of inflammation or change in liver function.

As with chronic hepatitis B virus infection, chronic infection with hepatitis C virus is associated with development of hepatocellular carcinoma (primary liver cancer). While almost all patients with chronic hepatitis C who develop cancer also have cirrhosis, cancer in non-cirrhotic livers has been reported. An important aspect of follow-up care for the chronically infected patient with hepatitis C virus is screening for hepatocellular carcinoma. There are no strict guidelines regarding frequency and no data exist on overall efficacy and cost-effectiveness of such screening. Patients with chronic hepatitis C should probably have periodic ultrasound tests to check for small liver masses. Blood should also be tested periodically for alpha-fetoprotein, a marker for hepatocellular carcinoma. Patients with cirrhosis should probably have more frequent "cancer screenings" than patients without cirrhosis. Again, good data on the efficacy and cost effectiveness of cancer screening do not exist and it is up to the individual doctor to determine how frequently "periodic" screening should be performed.

Vaccination against hepatitis A and hepatitis B are recommended for individuals with chronic hepatitis C. Some studies have suggested that patients with chronic hepatitis C are at increased risk for developing fulminant hepatic failure as a result of hepatitis A virus infection compared to healthy individuals. Acute hepatitis B virus infection may also be more dangerous in someone having another chronic liver disease. For these reasons, vaccination against hepatitis A and B for individuals with chronic hepatitis C who are not immune to these other viral infections is indicated.

Hepatitis C virus–human immunodeficiency virus (HIV) co-infection

The modes of transmission of hepatitis C virus are the same as or similar to those for the human immunodeficiency virus (HIV). Co-infection with hepatitis C virus and HIV is not unusual. Co-infection with hepatitis B virus is also not uncommon and was discussed earlier in this book.

A detailed discussion of treatment options for HIV-hepatitis C virus co-infected patients is beyond the scope of this book. A great deal depends upon the particular case and the doctor's judgment. In general, patients with HIV infection but a healthy immune system (normal CD4 or "T cell" counts) and no complications of AIDS who have hepatitis C infection should probably be treated the same as a patient without HIV infection. In early studies, patients with chronic hepatitis C and HIV co-infection generally did not respond well to treatment with interferon alpha. However, since the inception of routine treatment with protease inhibitors and combination therapy for HIV, patients are living much longer without signs of immune system deterioration. For this reason, treatment has to be reevaluated in this group of patients. Such studies are currently under way. In general, equally aggressive diagnostic procedures and treatments should be considered for patients with hepatitis C virus and HIV co-infection without laboratory evidence of a compromised immune system or clinical evidence of AIDS. In individuals with very low CD4 counts or with AIDS, a less aggressive approach to hepatitis C may be indicated as other problems may be more immediate. Again, the medical approach taken depends upon the individual case and the doctor's judgment.

Prevention

Hepatitis C is a contagious disease. All individuals infected with hepatitis C are potentially contagious and should be considered as such. Several precautionary measures can prevent the spread of hepatitis C. Many of the following recommendations for prevention can be found in the National Institutes of Health's Consensus Development Statement on Hepatitis C. Others have been made by the U.S. Centers for Disease Control and Prevention.

In the health care setting, adherence to universal (standard) precautions for the protection of medical personnel and patients is essential. Patients known to be infected with hepatitis C virus should not donate blood and, in most cases, should not be organ donors (a possible exception may be to donate an organ to someone with chronic hepatitis C). People living in the same house as an individual infected with hepatitis C should use common sense about exposure to blood and blood products. They should not share razors or toothbrushes. Covering open wounds is recommended. Injection needles, which may be in the home if they are used to administer interferon alpha, should be disposed of carefully using standard precautionary techniques. It is not necessary to avoid close contact with family members or sharing meals or utensils. There is no evidence that hepatitis C is spread by casual contact such as hand-holding, hugging, or kissing. There is probably less than a 5 percent risk of a pregnant mother transmitting hepatitis C virus to her newborn baby. There is no evidence at this time that hepatitis C virus is transmitted by breast feeding.

Regarding sexual transmission, the recommendations for prevention differ for individuals with multiple partners and those in long-term monogamous relationships. For individuals with multiple sex partners, latex condoms should be used by men with hepatitis C or by the male partners of female patients. On the other hand, according to the U.S. Centers for Disease Control and Prevention, it is not recommended to change sexual practices for individuals in long-term monogamous relationships if one partner has chronic hepatitis C.

At the present time, there is no effective vaccine for hepatitis C, and it does not look as if one will be available in the near future. Problems in vaccine development include the existence of various genotypes of the hepatitis C virus and the ability of the virus to mutate and form quasispecies. Additional research will hopefully lead to the development of an effective treatment against hepatitis C.

Hepatitis D

Definition and symptoms

The hepatitis D virus is a small circular RNA virus also referred to as hepatitis delta virus and classified in the family Deltaviridae. The hepatitis D virus is replication defective and cannot propagate in the absence of another virus. In humans, *hepatitis D virus infection occurs only in the presence of hepatitis B virus infection;* in other words, it *cannot* infect individuals unless they also have hepatitis B.

The hepatitis D virus causes acute and chronic hepatitis in individuals infected with the hepatitis B virus. It should be suspected either in individuals who have chronic hepatitis B and a sudden worsening in condition, or in those who present with very severe acute hepatitis B. In *co-infection,* a person is infected with both the hepatitis B virus and hepatitis D virus *at the same time.* Persons with co-infection may present with a more severe acute disease and higher risk of fulminant hepatic failure compared to those infected with hepatitis B virus alone. Co-infection usually results in acute hepatitis. Adults who are co-infected with both the hepatitis D virus and hepatitis B virus are *less* likely to develop chronic hepatitis B than those infected with hepatitis B virus alone.

In *superinfection,* an individual already infected with the hepatitis B virus becomes infected with hepatitis D virus. This might occur in a drug user who already has chronic hepatitis B and continues to inject drugs. Superinfection with the hepatitis D virus may be associated with a sudden worsening of liver disease and symptoms such as jaundice. The blood ALT and AST activities may become more elevated. Individuals with chronic hepatitis B who are superinfected with hepatitis D virus usually become chronically infected with hepatitis D virus, too. The risk of developing cirrhosis is greater in individuals chronically infected with both the hepatitis B and hepatitis D viruses compared to those infected with hepatitis B virus alone. As many as 80 percent of individuals chronically infected with both of these viruses may ultimately develop cirrhosis.

Transmission

The hepatitis D virus is transmitted in ways similar to the hepatitis B virus. One mode of transmission is intravenous drug use. Transmission from multiple blood transfusions is also possible but screening of the blood supply for hepatitis B virus also eliminates the hepatitis D virus. Sexual transmission of the hepatitis D virus is less efficient than for the hepatitis B virus. Although hepatitis D virus can be transmitted from mothers to their newborn babies, transmission by this route is rare.

The global distribution of hepatitis D virus infection is similar to that for hepatitis B virus. In some parts of the world, such as southern Italy and Russia, hepatitis D virus infection is fairly common among individuals chronically infected with hepatitis B. It is found in about 20 percent of so-called chronic carriers and as many as 60 percent of individuals with clinical hepatitis caused by hepatitis B virus. In northern Italy, Spain, and Egypt, about 10 percent of asymptomatic "chronic carriers" infected with hepatitis B, and about 30 to 50 percent of symptomatic patients with hepatitis B, are infected with the hepatitis D virus. In most of China and other parts of southeast Asia where the prevalence of chronic hepatitis B virus infection approaches 10 percent of the entire population, hepatitis D virus infection is rare.

Diagnosis

Diagnosis of hepatitis D virus infection is determined by blood testing. In acute co-infection, IgM and IgG antibodies to hepatitis D virus are detectable during the course of infection. IgM antibodies will be detected earlier after acute infection and IgG later or while the patient is recovering. IgG antibody concentrations in blood generally fall to levels that cannot be detected until after the acute infection resolves. There is no reliable marker that persists to indicate past infection with hepatitis D virus. In hepatitis D virus superinfection, high levels of both IgM and IgG antibodies against the hepatitis D virus become detectable after infection. Both IgM and IgG antibodies persist in serum as long as the patient remains infected.

Hepatitis D virus co-infection often is not diagnosed. In cases in which acute hepatitis B is not too severe, the doctor will not search for hepatitis D co-infection. If liver disease is un-usually severe in a high-risk individual, testing for antibodies against hepatitis D virus may be performed and the diagnosis of acute co-infection made. In chronic hepatitis D, which occurs usually as superinfection, the presence of IgG antibodies in blood against hepatitis D virus, in a patient with detectable blood HBsAg, establishes the diagnosis. Testing will usually be performed in a patient with known chronic hepatitis B whose condition deteriorates.

Tests for IgG against hepatitis D virus are commercially available in the U.S. Tests for IgM antibodies are available only in research laboratories. Tests for a hepatitis D virus protein known as hepatitis D antigen and PCR tests for hepatitis D virus RNA are also available in research laboratories. They are not part of routine diagnostic testing, however. Tests for hepatitis D antigen and viral RNA directly detect the presence of virus in the patient's blood.

Treatment

Treatment of acute hepatitis D virus co-infection is support-ive. Either the patient gets better spontaneously or develops ful-minant hepatic failure. Emergency liver transplantation is an option for fulminant hepatic failure. In chronic hepatitis D infec-tion, treatment with interferon alpha is a consideration. Although not much data are available at present, some studies suggest that higher doses of interferon alpha, such as 10 million units every day, are necessary in hepatitis D co-infection compared to the 5 million units used every day for chronic hepatitis B.

Prevention

Because the hepatitis D virus needs hepatitis B virus to repli-cate, co-infection can be prevented if hepatitis B virus infection is prevented. Patients immune to hepatitis B infection cannot get infected with the hepatitis D virus. Therefore, vaccination against hepatitis B virus will eliminate the chance of contracting hepatitis D. Universal vaccination for hepatitis B should, therefore, theoretically eliminate hepatitis D as a human disease.

Individuals not immune to hepatitis B infection, who have knowingly been exposed to the hepatitis B and hepatitis D viruses, can receive passive immunization with hepatitis B immune globulin (HBIG). Prevention of hepatitis B virus infection by HBIG will not permit hepatitis D virus infection. No vaccine exists to prevent hepatitis D virus superinfection of persons with chronic hepatitis B virus infection. In these cases, prevention rests entirely upon avoiding high-risk behaviors. As always, high-risk sexual activities should be avoided and latex condoms used. Intravenous drugs should not be used.

Hepatitis E

Definition and symptoms

The hepatitis E virus is a small, spherical virus that has been provisionally classified as a member of the Caliciviridae family. It is possible that this family assignment will change because the hepatitis E viral genome is different than that of most other caliciviruses. Its genome is composed of RNA.

The hepatitis E virus causes only acute liver disease. The disease caused by hepatitis E virus infection is known as hepatitis E. Hepatitis E is very similar to hepatitis A in its symptoms and clinical course. The disease can range from extremely mild to fulminant hepatic failure. Some cases of acute infection with hepatitis E virus may not produce any symptoms at all and go undiagnosed. In most hepatitis E outbreaks, the highest rates of clinically evident hepatitis have occurred in young to middle-age adults. It is possible that infected children, as is the case with hepatitis A, are more likely to have no obvious disease after infection. The time from infection to symptoms varies from fifteen to sixty days with forty days being the average. It is not yet clear when the greatest danger of infecting others occurs, but virus excretion in feces has been demonstrated up to fourteen days after acute illness.

Patients with relatively mild disease may suffer from nausea, vomiting, fever, fatigue, and loss of appetite. Blood tests may reveal elevations in ALT and AST activities and possibly elevations in bilirubin concentration. Patients with more severe disease may develop jaundice and blood tests will reveal an elevation in bilirubin concentration, a prolongation of prothrombin time, and sometimes markedly elevated ALT and AST activities. Most patients with mild or moderate hepatitis E recover without complications. Some patients become so sick that they cannot eat or drink. Some patients with hepatitis E infection develop fulminant hepatic failure.

Transmission

Hepatitis E virus infection does not occur in the U.S. Virtually all cases reported in the U.S. have affected travelers returning from parts of the world where hepatitis E is common. Outbreaks have occurred in many geographic locations around the world, mostly in underdeveloped countries. Hepatitis E virus is primarily spread by the fecal-oral route, that is, from feces of infected individuals to food or water that is then ingested by others. Drinking of contaminated water is probably the most common mode of infection. Person-to-person transmission appears to be rare. Like hepatitis A, hepatitis E is more common in parts of the world having poor sanitary conditions. Travelers from developed countries to such regions are at increased risk for infection from hepatitis E.

Diagnosis

The clinical diagnosis of hepatitis E infection is suggested by the sudden onset of liver disease fifteen to sixty days after suspected exposure to hepatitis E. Typically, patients will present with symptoms including fever, nausea, vomiting, loss of appetite, and fatigue. Sometimes, patients will present with new onset jaundice immediately suggesting acute liver disease. Such patients should be questioned about a risk factor for hepatitis E, which in North America and most European countries is recent travel to an area where the disease is endemic. Southern and central Asia, northern Africa, and Central America are regions of the world where hepatitis E outbreaks are the most common.

The diagnosis of hepatitis E infection is made through blood testing. Tests for antibodies against the hepatitis E virus are not commercially available in the U.S. but are available at research laboratories or specialized centers, such as the Centers for Disease Control and Prevention in Atlanta, Georgia. Both IgM and IgG antibodies against the hepatitis E virus are elicited following acute viral infection. IgM antibodies disappear as the patient recovers and is the best test to diagnose acute disease. IgG antibodies persist for some period of time after infection and may provide protection against recurrent infection. In addition to testing for antibodies in the blood, other tests for hepatitis E infection are available on a research basis in the U.S. PCR tests can detect hepatitis E virus RNA in blood or stool during infection. Tests to detect viral proteins in blood and liver are also available in some research laboratories.

Treatment

There is no specific treatment for hepatitis E. In most cases, the disease is mild and self-limiting. If the patient is so sick that he or she cannot eat or drink, hospitalization may be necessary for the administration of intravenous fluids. The patient can be discharged once there is adequate oral intake. In serious cases, generally those causing fulminant hepatic failure, hospitalization and intensive care are required. Preferably, these patients should be hospitalized in a medical center where liver transplantation can be performed if necessary.

Prevention

The most important issue regarding hepatitis E is prevention. Prevention of hepatitis E depends primarily upon avoiding contaminated water. Travelers to developing countries should avoid drinking from local water supplies and consuming beverages with ice of unknown purity. Uncooked shellfish, uncooked fruits, and vegetables that are not peeled or prepared by the traveler should not be consumed. At the present time, there are no postexposure prophylactic measures nor vaccines for hepatitis E.

Hepatitis G?

In 1995 and 1996, three novel RNA viruses were identified as members of the Flaviviridae family and shown to be somewhat similar to the hepatitis C virus. These three viruses were termed GB-A, GB-B, and GB-C by workers who discovered them at Abbott Laboratories. The genetic material of the GB-A and GB-B viruses was isolated from the blood of a tamarin (a species of monkey) infected with the blood of a surgeon with initials GB who died from what appeared to be, at the time, non-A, non-B hepatitis. Subsequent work determined that these two viruses are likely tamarin viruses that do not infect humans. Based on genetic information about GB-A and GB-B viruses, the investigators who discovered them isolated the genetic material of a related virus they called GB-C from the blood of a human with chronic hepatitis.

Concurrent with the discovery of the GB-C virus, another group at Genelabs Technologies discovered a virus they called hepatitis G virus. They identified the virus in blood from a patient with chronic hepatitis C. They ultimately discovered that the genetic material of this virus was different than that of the hepatitis C virus. It was the same as that of the GB-C discovered by workers at Abbott Laboratories.

The hepatitis G/GB-C virus appears to infect humans and it is present in the blood supply. It seems to be transmitted by blood and blood products. However, most investigators now think that the hepatitis G/GB-C virus does *not* cause meaningful liver disease. The general feeling is that the hepatitis G/GB-C virus is an "innocent bystander" that can infect humans but not cause disease.

Due to their similar modes of transmission, the hepatitis G/GB-C virus is often found in patients who are already infected with hepatitis C virus. These individuals do not appear to do any worse than those infected with only hepatitis C. At the present time, there is probably no reason to test patients for infection with the hepatitis G/GB-C virus. This recommendation may change should it ever be clearly established that it can cause liver disease. Testing for hepatitis G/GB-C virus in blood by PCR is available commercially at some clinical laboratories.

Other Viruses that Cause Hepatitis

Hepatitis A, B, C, D, and E viruses are the major hepatotropic viruses that cause liver disease in humans (there is no hepatitis F). Some other viruses can also cause acute liver disease in otherwise healthy individuals. In most cases, these viruses cause systemic diseases that concurrently affect the liver. These viruses included dengue virus, yellow fever virus, and Epstein-Barr virus (EBV), which causes mononucleosis. Individuals with mononucleosis can suffer from a mild form of acute hepatitis that always resolves. Available data suggest that pox virus and measles virus may cause chronic hepatitis in children.

Some viruses that are generally harmless in healthy individuals may cause liver disease in patients with compromised immune systems. These viruses may infect patients with AIDS or cancer. They may also infect patients who have received organ transplants and are taking medications that suppress their immune systems. The most important of these viruses is cytomegalovirus or CMV. Cytomegalovirus can cause hepatitis in recipients of organ transplants, including transplanted livers. CMV can also cause hepatitis and serious bile duct abnormalities in patients with AIDS.

Some doctors will test patients with chronic hepatitis for antibodies against CMV and EBV. These viruses are endemic in the human population and the detection of IgG antibodies means virtually nothing. Furthermore, these two viruses do not cause any significant chronic liver disease in people with normal immune systems. If someone tells you that you have chronic hepatitis caused by EBV or CMV, you should be suspicious.

Fatty Liver

Definition and Symptoms

Fatty liver and *steatosis* are terms used to describe a pathological observation and not a disease per se. In response to various insults, fat accumulates in the hepatocytes in either large droplets (macrovesicular) or tiny little droplets (microvesicular). This can readily be seen on liver biopsy. Some of the insults that cause fat accumulation in hepatocytes are listed in Table 4.11.

Although, strictly speaking, it is a pathological diagnosis, the term *fatty liver* is frequently used to refer to a clinical entity. Generally, it is used to describe what would be diagnosed by a

Table 4.11. *Causes of steatosis or fatty liver.*

Macrovesicular steatosis	Excessive alcohol consumption
	Obesity
	Diabetes mellitus
	Malnutrition
	Elevated blood triglycerides (cause of or result of?)
	After intestinal bypass surgery
	Total parenteral nutrition
	Idiopathic (cause not known)
Microvesicular steatosis	Reye syndrome
	Fatty liver of pregnancy
	Sometimes with excessive alcohol consumption
	Drugs (common ones include tetracycline and valproic acid)
	Rare inherited metabolic diseases
	Jamaican vomiting sickness (caused by a toxin from the unripened fruit of the ackee tree)

pathologist as macrovesicular steatosis and not attributable to alcohol. Patients usually do *not* have symptoms or physical signs of liver disease. Abnormalities usually detected by routine blood tests, or tests performed to evaluate other conditions, are usually the first indications of fatty liver. Patients with fatty liver are usually, but not always, obese and/or diabetic.

Diagnosis

When a patient is found to have elevated ALT and AST activities in blood tests, the first questions asked usually concern alcohol use. The initial appropriate blood tests are for hepatitis B surface antigen and antibodies against the hepatitis C virus to exclude chronic viral hepatitis. If investigation reveals no history of excessive alcohol consumption and no evidence of hepatitis B or hepatitis C virus infection, fatty liver is often suspected. Drugs, metabolic disorders, and autoimmune hepatitis should also be excluded as possibilities where appropriate. The diagnosis is more strongly suspected in individuals who are obese or have diabetes mellitus.

Many doctors will perform an ultrasound examination on patients with elevated blood ALT and AST activities even though there are few, if any, conditions that cause asymptomatic elevations in these lab tests that can be diagnosed by this procedure. Sometimes an ultrasound scan is reported to be "consistent with fatty infiltration of the liver." Fat has a different ultrasound density than normal liver tissue and the presence of fat in the liver can be *suggested by* ultrasound examination. However, the detection of fat density on ultrasound examination cannot clearly establish the presence of fat in hepatocytes. Furthermore, ultrasound cannot distinguish between steatosis and *steatohepatitis,* a type of inflammation associated with fat in hepatocytes. Furthermore, in patients with steatosis or steatohepatitis, the ultrasound examination will frequently be normal. Ultrasound, and for that matter CAT scan, are not reliable tests for the diagnosis of fatty liver. The diagnosis of fatty liver can be made only by liver biopsy.

Typically, "fatty liver" is suspected when:

1. The patient has elevated ALT and/or AST activities on blood tests.
2. The patient does not drink significant amounts of alcohol and does not take medications that can affect the liver.
3. The patient is usually (not always) obese and/or suffers from diabetes mellitus.

4. Hepatitis B and hepatitis C virus infections are reliably excluded by history and laboratory testing.
5. Metabolic and autoimmune liver diseases are unlikely based upon history and, if necessary, the results of laboratory testing.
6. An ultrasound examination is done and may or may not be consistent with fatty infiltration of the liver.

At this point, what will most doctors do? And what should be done? As in many other areas of medicine, there are no absolute right or wrong answers.

One important consideration is whether elevations in the blood ALT and/or AST activities have persisted for more than six months. In patients presenting for the first time with only modest elevations in the aminotransferase activities, when other causes of liver disease have already been reliably excluded, it is reasonable to perform repeat blood testing over the next six months. If physical examination and/or laboratory tests such as bilirubin, albumin, and prothrombin time suggest abnormal liver function, however, liver biopsy should probably be performed sooner.

What if the patient has had elevations in blood ALT and AST activities for six months or longer? If the diagnosis of fatty liver is strongly suspected on clinical grounds, for example, if the patient is obese and/or suffers from diabetes, many doctors will defer liver biopsy and say that the patient has "fatty liver." But as I have already mentioned, the diagnosis can be suspected but *not* diagnosed without a liver biopsy. For these reasons, most liver specialists would probably perform liver biopsies in patients suspected of having fatty liver to definitely establish the diagnosis.

Why is liver biopsy critical in the evaluation of patients with suspected fatty liver? First, it is the *only* way to establish the diagnosis. Second, it is necessary to exclude other possible conditions that were deemed to be unlikely based on history, physical examination, and laboratory testing. Even in patients in whom fatty liver is strongly suspected, another diagnosis will sometimes be discovered by liver biopsy. Third, *liver biopsy is the only way to distinguish between steatosis and steatohepatitis.* And this is a critical distinction. Steatohepatitis, which is often called *nonalcoholic steatohepatitis* or *NASH* if it is not caused by alcohol consumption, carries a worse prognosis than steatosis. Patients with steatosis probably do not have progressive liver disease. However, *NASH can progress to cirrhosis and can be diagnosed only by liver biopsy.* A doctor *cannot* state that you have NASH without doing a biopsy.

To summarize some of the major points about fatty liver and its diagnosis:

1. The most common causes of fatty liver (excluding excessive alcohol consumption) are obesity and diabetes mellitus. It can occur in individuals without these conditions, however.
2. Fatty liver can be suspected but not diagnosed without performing a liver biopsy.
3. Fatty liver can be definitively diagnosed only by liver biopsy.
4. The distinction between steatosis and steatohepatitis can be made only by liver biopsy.

Treatment

How is fatty liver treated? To the best of my knowledge, there are no prospective randomized studies that have established this. Based on clinical experience and common sense, however, it is likely that several reasonable interventions will "cure" or improve steatosis and steatohepatitis.

The basic approach to treatment is to remove the underlying cause of fatty infiltration of the liver and lessen exposure to things that can worsen it such as:

• Weight loss if obese or even if slightly overweight
• Better control of blood sugar if diabetic
• Low-fat diet
• Aerobic exercise
• Strictly limit or avoid alcohol

Patients who are obese, or even only slightly overweight, should lose weight. In the experience of many liver specialists, and in small observation studies, weight loss has been shown to improve fatty liver based upon return of blood ALT and AST activities to normal. Weight loss is best achieved by a combination of diet and exercise; either one alone will not be as efficient.

Even in patients who are not overweight, or once a patient reaches ideal body weight, a low-fat diet and exercise should be continued. People who have, or have had, fatty liver are likely predisposed to develop it. Therefore, such individuals should pay careful attention to maintaining a low fat intake and to "burning off" fats by aerobic exercise.

Alcohol is the major cause of fatty infiltration of the liver, and NASH appears identical to alcoholic hepatitis on liver biopsy. Common sense therefore dictates that patients with steatosis or steatohepatitis should limit alcohol intake, although there is no strict lower limit. Besides its direct effects on the liver, alcohol also contains needless calories that are best avoided. Patients with steatohepatitis should probably completely refrain from alcohol consumption. Although there are no studies to support it, the fact that steatohepatitis and alcoholic hepatitis look so similar strongly suggests that alcohol will worsen the condition.

Steatosis and steatohepatitis can be present in patients with diabetes mellitus, and diabetics whose blood sugars are less well controlled may be more likely to develop them. Tight control of blood sugars should therefore be attempted in diabetics with fatty liver.

Overall, the prognosis for most patients with fatty liver is quite good—from a strictly "liver point of view." However, steatohepatitis can lead to cirrhosis. And although no studies have proven this, steatosis *may* turn into steatohepatitis if the patient accumulates excess fat. Therefore, patients with steatosis should make the necessary lifestyle changes to prevent this from occurring.

Fatty liver (steatosis and steatohepatitis) is "treated" by maintaining an overall healthy lifestyle. Eating well, exercising, maintaining ideal body weight, and limiting alcohol intake will improve not only fatty liver but also, perhaps even more significantly, *overall* health. I often tell an obese patient with fatty liver thatsdf although the fat in the liver will probably not lead to significant liver disease, *"you should think about what excessive fat in your body will do to your heart."* Patients with fatty liver resulting from obesity and poorly controlled diabetes are at increased risk for serious diseases such as heart attack, stroke, and possibly cancer. Obese patients with fatty liver who lead unhealthy lifestyles should consider fatty liver a *warning sign* for development of other serious diseases. They should heed this warning and start living healthier lives.

Autoimmune Liver Diseases

Autoimmune diseases are those in which tissue injury is caused by the person's own immune system attacking the body. Some autoimmune diseases, such as systemic lupus erythematosus, are "systemic" in that many different organs are attacked. Others are relatively organ-specific, including the liver diseases we will discuss in this section.

The "causes" of most autoimmune diseases, including those that affect the liver, are not known. It is not entirely clear why an individual's immune system will, all of a sudden, attack constituents of his or, more often, her own body. There are very likely genetic factors that predispose people to develop autoimmune diseases. Mutations in certain genes in mice are associated with autoimmune diseases, and autoimmune diseases "tend" to run in families. However, autoimmune diseases are *not* strictly inherited and a relative of someone with one will *most likely not get the disease*. It is also possible that environmental factors trigger autoimmune diseases in individuals who are genetically predisposed.

Patients with autoimmune diseases may have very specific antibodies in their blood against proteins, fats, or DNA inside their own cells. Antibodies that recognize constituents of a person's own body are known as *autoantibodies*. The recognized constituents are sometimes called *autoantigens*. Autoantibodies are often classified based on the part of the cell in which their autoantigens are localized, for example, as antinuclear antibodies (ANA) or antimitochondrial antibodies (AMA). In most cases, it is not clear how, or if, autoantibodies and the autoantigens they recognize contribute to the disease process. Nonetheless, disease-specific autoantibodies have found tremendous utility as reliable diagnostic markers, even if they do not cause the disease being diagnosed. Blood testing for autoantibodies therefore often plays a critical role in the diagnosis of autoimmune diseases.

Three major liver diseases are considered autoimmune: autoimmune hepatitis, primary biliary cirrhosis (PBC), and primary sclerosing cholangitis (PSC). In autoimmune hepatitis, the immune response is directed against the hepatocytes and the clinical picture is that of hepatitis. In PBC, the immune response is directed against the smallest bile ducts within the liver and the clinical picture is related to their inflammation and obstruction. In PSC, the immune response is against the larger bile ducts inside and outside the liver and the illness manifests with symptoms attributable to bile duct obstruction.

Autoimmune Hepatitis

Definition and symptoms

Autoimmune hepatitis was first described as "lupoid" hepatitis. This term should no longer be used. The term *lupoid* is additionally confusing because there is no relationship between autoimmune hepatitis and systemic lupus erythematosus. Autoimmune hepatitis affects primarily women. About 80 percent of affected individuals are women, usually between the ages of fifteen and forty. More rarely, autoimmune hepatitis affects both much older and much younger individuals.

Although it is a chronic disease, many patients first present to medical attention acutely ill with jaundice, fever, symptoms of severe liver dysfunction, and a picture that sometimes resembles fulminant hepatic failure. Other patients may first come to medical attention because of nonspecific symptoms or blood test abnormalities suggestive of chronic hepatitis. In addition to liver disease, some patients with autoimmune hepatitis also suffer from fever, joint aches, muscle pains, fluid accumulation in various parts of the body, and low platelet counts. Other patients already have cirrhosis when they are first diagnosed with autoimmune hepatitis. If left untreated (or if it does not respond to therapy), autoimmune hepatitis can lead to severe liver failure before cirrhosis develops. Such patients may suffer from hepatitis for several months, or even weeks, and then develop liver failure and need liver transplantation to survive.

Diagnosis

Diagnosis of autoimmune hepatitis is made based upon a combination of clinical, laboratory, immunological, and pathological criteria. Autoimmune hepatitis should be suspected in any young patient—especially a woman—with clinical evidence of hepatitis. It should be suspected especially in individuals not abusing alcohol, not taking drugs, with no family history of metabolic liver disease, and without evidence of viral hepatitis. Patients usually present with moderate to severe hepatitis; their ALT and AST activities are elevated on blood tests. Some patients with relatively mild liver inflammation may have only laboratory abnormalities as their initial presentation. In some instances, patients with autoimmune hepatitis first present to doctors or emergency rooms with severe liver failure and hepatic encephalopathy that closely resembles fulminant hepatic failure. The blood ALT and AST activities will usually be markedly elevated, the bilirubin concentration high in these patients, and the prothrombin time prolonged.

Serum protein electrophoresis and testing for autoantibodies are of central importance in the diagnosis of autoimmune hepatitis. Patients with one type of autoimmune hepatitis (type I) have gamma-globulin concentrations more than twice normal and sometimes antinuclear antibodies and/or antismooth muscle antibodies in their blood. Patients with another type of autoimmune hepatitis (type II) may have normal or only slightly elevated gamma-globulin concentrations but have antibodies against a particular cytochrome p450 protein that are called anti-LKM (liver kidney microsome) antibodies. Patients with yet another type (type III) have autoantibodies called anti-SLA (soluble liver antigen) antibodies. This classification of autoimmune hepatitis into types I, II, and III is not really that important to patients; what is important to realize is that special blood tests for autoantibodies and gamma-globulin concentration are central to the diagnosis.

Patients in whom a diagnosis of autoimmune hepatitis is suspected should have a liver biopsy. If immediate liver biopsy is contraindicated because of a prolonged prothrombin time or low platelet count, treatment (see below) should be started prior to biopsy if the diagnosis is likely based on clinical and laboratory criteria (for example, a young woman with severe hepatitis, an elevated blood gamma-globulin concentration, and negative risk factors and blood tests for viral hepatitis). The patient will often improve rapidly with treatment, and biopsy should be performed to confirm the diagnosis when the prothrombin time and platelet count return to safe ranges. Certain features on liver biopsy strongly support the diagnosis of autoimmune hepatitis. In addition, liver biopsy is usually the only way to know with certainty if a patient with autoimmune hepatitis has cirrhosis.

A scoring system for diagnosis of autoimmune has been devised in which certain diagnostic features are given points depending upon how suggestive they are for autoimmune hepatitis. Features with positive points include female sex, the presence of certain autoantibodies, a high concentration of blood and gamma-globulin, and certain findings on biopsy. Examples of diagnostic features given negative points are laboratory evidence of hepatitis C virus or hepatitis B virus infection. When these diagnostic features are scored and totaled, the diagnosis of autoimmune hepatitis is classified as either unlikely, probable, or likely. It is not important for patients to know the details of the scoring system but to realize that clinical judgment and several different investigative measures are considered together in making the diagnosis. *There is no one test for the diagnosis of autoimmune hepatitis.*

Treatment

Steroids, usually prednisone or prednisolone, and azathioprine (Imuran) form the cornerstones of treatment for autoimmune hepatitis. These drugs suppress the immune system. Once the doctor is confident about the diagnosis, treatment should be started immediately. Some doctors start prednisone or prednisolone alone and others start azathioprine along with one of these. Usually, the steroid dose is higher if used alone.

About three-quarters of patients with autoimmune hepatitis respond rapidly to treatment based on improvement in symptoms and laboratory test results. Repeat liver biopsy, if performed, usually indicates tremendous resolution of inflammation. Once a patient responds, the steroid and/or azathioprine should be gradually tapered to the lowest possible dose that keeps ALT and AST activities normal or very near normal. Unfortunately, some patients will not have a good response to treatment no matter how much medication is used. Experimental therapies in the setting of approved clinical trials may be appropriate for these individuals.

Maintaining a patient on the lowest doses of prednisone and/or azathioprine to keep the disease under control is usually more trial and error than precise science. In some patients, all medications can be stopped after several months of treatment and the patient will not need any to keep ALT and AST normal. However, such patients can "relapse" and again have clinical or laboratory evidence of liver inflammation in the future. In other patients, a low dose of steroid, azathioprine, or a combination of both is necessary to keep disease activity under control. Some patients have a fluctuating course in which blood ALT activities increase and decrease over time. These patients may need slightly more medication at certain times to keep liver inflammation minimal and slightly less medication at other times. For these reasons, all patients with autoimmune hepatitis should have follow-up visits regularly with a doctor experienced in treating this disease.

Over the long term, most patients with autoimmune hepatitis will develop cirrhosis despite having a response to treatment. Nonetheless, treatment is essential as the progression of disease can be rapid and dramatic without it. Treatment will significantly slow the progression to cirrhosis. Even patients who already have cirrhosis at presentation should be treated because stopping the inflammation will halt ongoing liver damage and the rapid development of complications or liver failure. For patients with chronic autoimmune hepatitis who develop complications of cirrhosis or liver failure, liver transplantation is an effective procedure. The disease almost never recurs in the transplanted liver, possibly due in part to powerful drugs used to suppress the immune system to prevent transplant rejection.

Primary Biliary Cirrhosis

Definition and symptoms

Primary biliary cirrhosis is generally referred to by doctors and patients as *PBC*. The disease was first described in the 1950s. Primary biliary cirrhosis is actually a misnomer for this disease. The defining abnormality in PBC is *not* biliary cirrhosis, which is a general term meaning cirrhosis resulting from bile duct disorders. However, after many years of having the disease, patients almost invariably end up with biliary cirrhosis. The defining pathological abnormality in PBC is inflammation of the smallest bile ducts in the liver. Dr. Hans Popper and Dr. Fenton Schaffner, who performed one of the first detailed pathological characterizations of PBC in the 1960s, proposed the name "non-suppurative cholangitis" for this disease. This is a much better description of the characteristic pathological lesion of PBC that means inflammation of the bile duct (cholangitis) without pus (non-suppurative). Unfortunately, this term never caught on, and primary biliary cirrhosis, or PBC, is the term now used by everyone.

PBC occurs worldwide but its exact prevalence is not clear. Estimates are that about 150 to 240 of every million people have PBC. The problem with population studies is that the disease is often not diagnosed accurately by many doctors in different parts of the world. One thing is certain about who gets PBC: *mostly women*. Ninety percent of those with PBC are female.

PBC is diagnosed usually in middle-aged women. The disease is not always immediately suspected by their examining doctors, and presentation can vary. Very often, individuals with early PBC have few or no symptoms. Sometimes, patients will not see doctors until they have complications of cirrhosis. The most typical presentations are similar to the following three hypothetical cases:

CASE 1. A forty-year-old woman has been suffering from itching all over her body for the past several weeks. There is no rash. Various creams and over-the-counter remedies have not helped. She sees her doctor, who also cannot readily explain the itching. The doctor prescribes an antihistamine that still does not help. The patient returns a couple of weeks later with self-inflicted scratch marks all over her body. Before referring the patient to a dermatologist, her doctor performs several blood tests and finds the alkaline phosphatase activity to be markedly elevated. An ultrasound examination of the liver is performed that is normal. The patient is referred to a gastroenterologist who does a blood test for antimitochondrial antibodies, which comes back positive. A liver biopsy is performed that is consistent with PBC.

CASE 2. A forty-five-year-old woman who appears completely healthy, is found to have elevated alkaline phosphatase and GGTP activities on "routine" blood tests by her gynecologist. The gynecologist refers the patient to an internist who makes a provisional diagnosis of PBC based on clinical history and laboratory testing. She is then referred to a liver specialist who performs a liver biopsy that confirms the diagnosis.

CASE 3. A fifty-seven-year-old woman who has seen a doctor regularly for many years due to high blood pressure now presents to an emergency room complaining of increasing abdominal girth and yellow eyes. The emergency room doctor discovers ascites and finds blood bilirubin concentration and alkaline phosphatase activity to be elevated. The patient is admitted to the hospital for further evaluation. A keen young medical student assigned to her case orders all the right tests to make a provisional diagnosis of PBC (and the medical student later graduates with honors). A liver biopsy shows biliary cirrhosis.

The most common presentations of patients with PBC are similar to those described in cases 1 and 2. A very typical presentation is that of a woman between the ages of forty and sixty who sees a doctor because of excessive itching (the medical term for itching is *pruritus*). Cholestasis, or stagnation of bile in the bile ducts in the liver, is associated with retention in the body of unknown factors that can cause itching. The retained factor in the blood responsible for the itching is not bilirubin as itching can occur with normal blood bilirubin concentration.

Another very typical presentation of PBC is that of a woman who has no complaints at all in whom elevated alkaline phosphatase activity is discovered on blood tests taken for other reasons. There are also less common presentations of PBC.

Sometimes, the patient does not see a doctor until the disease is fairly advanced. When the disease is more advanced, patients may see a doctor because of jaundice, or because of complications of cirrhosis such as ascites (as did the patient described in case 3). "Extra-hepatic," or symptoms not related to the liver, are also sometimes experienced by individuals with PBC. Dry eyes and dry mouth, known in medical jargon as *sicca syndrome* or *Sjögren syndrome,* is a frequent complaint. Various rashes and other skin abnormalities sometimes occur. Bone loss or *osteoporosis* is also frequently experienced by women with PBC.

PBC is an invariably progressive disease that leads to cirrhosis and ultimately end-stage liver disease. All patients diagnosed with this disease will either develop cirrhosis or die of something else first. What is difficult to predict is the rate of progression to cirrhosis or liver failure in a given patient. Some patients will progress to end-stage cirrhosis just a few years after diagnosis, while others will not develop cirrhosis for twenty years or more. This variability may be due in part to the fact that patients may have the disease without symptoms for a number of years before being diagnosed. Predicting the progression of disease in a patient with PBC is critically important because it allows the doctor to know when referral for liver transplantation is necessary.

Several complex mathematical equations have been devised to predict the progression of patients with PBC. Perhaps the most famous is the so-called Mayo equation. These equations consider a wide range of laboratory parameters, symptoms, physical signs, and biopsy findings. Of all the parameters in these equations, the blood bilirubin concentration is probably the best predictor of disease progression if complications of cirrhosis that predict a rapidly deteriorating course are not yet present. Once the blood bilirubin concentration exceeds 6 mg per deciliter, the patient's life expectancy is about two years. Patients with rising bilirubin concentrations should be referred for liver transplant evaluation.

Diagnosis

Diagnosis of PBC depends upon a combination of historical, laboratory, immunological, and liver biopsy data. There is usually no one test that will definitively diagnose PBC. In rare cases, a unique lesion of lymphocytic cells attacking a small bile duct can be seen on liver biopsy that is diagnostic. In general, the liver biopsy is *consistent with* PBC but not conclusively diagnostic.

Clinical criteria are important in diagnosing PBC. If clinical signs and symptoms are not compatible, the diagnosis should be suspect. A diagnosis of PBC in a man also deserves careful scrutiny, but it can occur. Other conditions that can cause biliary disease, including drugs, should be excluded by history.

Blood tests virtually always indicate elevations in alkaline phosphatase and GGTP activities. The AST and ALT activities are usually normal or only slightly above normal. The bilirubin and albumin concentrations and prothrombin time are normal early in the course and become abnormal as the disease progresses.

Immunological tests are of central importance to the diagnosis of PBC. More than 90 percent of patients will have *antimitochondrial antibodies* or *AMA* in their blood. These antibodies recognize proteins in mitochondria, which are tiny membrane-bound organelles found in all cells. In the clinical laboratory, these autoantibodies are detected by a type of microscopy in which the part of the cell that contains the recognized autoantigen can be identified. This test is pretty good for detection of antimitochondrial antibodies, but, in rare cases, it is falsely positive in patients who actually do not have them. In addition, some patients with diseases other than PBC have antibodies against different proteins in mitochondria.

About 10 percent or less of patients with PBC do not have detectable antimitochondrial antibodies on blood testing. These patients are sometimes said to have "AMA-negative PBC" or "autoimmune cholangitis." If all other aspects of the history, laboratory test results, and liver biopsy findings point to the diagnosis, patients who are "AMA-negative" probably have PBC. Patients with PBC but without detectable antimitochondrial antibodies should not be considered as having some sort of special or distinct variant. It has *not* been demonstrated that so-called autoimmune cholangitis is a different disease than PBC.

In addition to antimitochondrial antibodies, about 50 percent of patients with PBC will have autoantibodies against nuclei (*antinuclear antibodies* or *ANA*). Except for certain antinuclear antibodies detected only in research laboratories, the presence of ANA are *not* specific for the diagnosis of PBC and are found in a variety of autoimmune diseases; sometimes even in normal individuals. Their presence in the blood supports but does not make definitive the diagnosis of PBC.

Over 90 percent of patients with PBC have an elevation in the total IgM antibody concentration in their blood. This is not specific for PBC, but if present in someone with other criteria suggestive of the disease, an elevated blood IgM concentration strongly supports the diagnosis. The absence of an elevated IgM concentration should make any doctor question the diagnosis of PBC, but it does not exclude it.

An important aspect of the *diagnostic* evaluation of PBC is liver biopsy. As mentioned above, the liver biopsy is rarely definitively diagnostic for PBC. However, a diagnosis based on clinical, laboratory, and immunological parameters is strongly supported by a *consistent* biopsy. Pathologists will usually "stage" the liver biopsy in PBC. A stage 1 biopsy is the *florid bile duct lesion* of lymphocytic white blood cells attacking a small bile duct that is diagnostic for PBC. This lesion is usually not seen. A stage 2 biopsy in PBC shows *ductular proliferation* or many abnormal small bile ducts. A stage 3 biopsy in PBC shows *fibrosis* and a stage 4 biopsy shows *biliary cirrhosis.* In general, the stages of the biopsy show a continuum of disease, from the least advanced (stage 1) to the most advanced (stage 4). As PBC can affect the liver in a nonuniform fashion, sometimes you will see two or more stages on the same biopsy, for example, ductular proliferation, or stage 2, and fibrosis, or stage 3. The stage of the biopsy in PBC correlates roughly to the rate of disease progression. It is not a precise predictor, however, and there are other criteria that better predict a patient's rate of progression to end-stage liver disease.

In sum, the diagnosis of PBC is made by a combination of clinical, laboratory, immunological, and biopsy criteria. There is rarely one diagnostic test result. Supreme Court Associate Justice Potter Stewart once said in an opinion on a case involving pornography: "I know it when I see it." The same can be said by an experienced liver specialist about PBC.

Treatment

Ursodiol (Actigall® or Urso®), a bile acid, has been shown to improve the blood test results and clinical symptoms in patients with PBC. The results of some studies also indicate that ursodiol slows progression of the disease. Ursodiol is not a "cure" for PBC, but it may significantly slow disease progression. It is a very safe drug with few side effects. For these reasons, all patients with PBC should probably receive ursodiol as there are benefits and the attendant risks are low. The recommended dose for patients with PBC is 13 to 15 mg per kilogram of body weight a day. Despite extensive study, no other medical therapies have been shown to conclusively slow progression of PBC. Notably, steroids may be detrimental. Other drugs, such as cyclosporin A and methotrexate, are being investigated in clinical trials.

Osteoporosis (loss of bone) is a common complication of PBC. This results, in part, from bile duct damage that causes decreased absorption of fat-soluble vitamins including vitamin D, which is necessary for adequate calcium absorption and bone formation. Patients with PBC, most of whom are women and at a generally increased risk for development of osteoporosis, should probably take supplemental calcium and multivitamins that include vitamin D to prevent bone loss. There are no serious risks to this treatment, and it may reduce osteoporosis which, in later life, can be devastating.

Pruritus (itching) can be incapacitating in some patients with PBC. This condition often responds to treatment with a bile acid-binding resin such as cholestyramine. This is a powder mixed with water and consumed as a suspension. If itching does not respond to treatment with cholestyramine, some studies suggest that opioid antagonists (drugs that counter the affects of opiates) such as naloxone or naltrexone may help.

Patients with PBC must realize that the disease invariably progresses, sometimes over a time period of many years. Most younger individuals will probably require liver transplantation at some time in their lives barring better treatments being developed. Older patients may die with, but not from, PBC. Liver transplantation is remarkably effective for patients with PBC. The key is for the doctor to refer the patient for transplantation at the correct time. Anyone with complications of cirrhosis such as ascites or bleeding esophageal varices should be referred to a transplantation center for evaluation. Most patients, however, do not develop these complications until late in the course of disease. As mentioned above, one of the best predictors of progression is blood bilirubin concentration. Once total bilirubin concentration in the blood begins to rise, probably by the time it reaches 4 mg per deciliter, the patient should be referred for liver transplant evaluation. As in all chronic liver disease, no single parameter substitutes for follow-up by an experienced specialist.

Primary Sclerosing Cholangitis

Definition and symptoms

Primary sclerosing cholangitis is often referred to as PSC. It is a chronic liver disease characterized by inflammation, destruction, and fibrosis of the large bile ducts within the liver, as well as the bile ducts outside the liver. The cause of PSC is unknown, but most investigators agree that it is an autoimmune disease. Other causes, such as infectious agents, toxins, or recurrent infections of the bile ducts, have not been absolutely excluded. PSC's worldwide prevalence is approximately 3 in 100,000 individuals. In contrast to PBC and autoimmune hepatitis and most other autoimmune diseases that primarily affect women, about 70 percent of patients with PSC are men. The strong association of PSC with inflammatory bowel disease also suggests it is an autoimmune disorder. About 75 percent of patients with PSC have inflammatory bowel disease, mainly ulcerative colitis.

Inflammation of the larger bile ducts in PSC can lead to strictures, or "narrowing." Sometimes, bile can get plugged in these strictures resulting in acute and almost complete blockage of bile flow. In such instances, patients will develop jaundice. These recurrent bouts of bile duct obstruction, along with destruction of bile ducts within the liver, eventually lead to biliary cirrhosis in most patients. Patients with PSC also often have recurrent episodes of *bacterial cholangitis,* which is an infection of the bile ducts with bacteria. Patients with bacterial cholangitis often have jaundice, fever, and right upper quadrant abdominal pain. In some patients, recurrent episodes of bacterial cholangitis, which can be fatal, are a very significant problem before cirrhosis develops. In other patients, bacterial cholangitis is not a frequent problem. Patients with PSC also bear an increased risk of cholangiocarcinoma or primary bile duct cancer. The average survival, or time until liver transplantation, in patients with PSC is around ten years from time of diagnosis.

Diagnosis

Many patients with PSC are diagnosed by discovering elevated alkaline phosphatase and GGTP activities in blood tests taken for other reasons. This testing may be part of an evaluation for inflammatory bowel disease, from which most patients with PSC also suffer. Some patients present with itching (pruritus), jaundice, fatigue, fever, weight loss, or signs of complications from cirrhosis. Others present for the first time with signs and symptoms of bacterial cholangitis such as fever, chills, and right upper quadrant abdominal pain.

Blood tests for PSC virtually always indicate elevated alkaline phosphatase and GGTP activities with lesser or no elevations in the aminotransferase activities. Early in the course of disease, the bilirubin concentration is usually normal or slightly elevated but it becomes markedly elevated late in the course of disease. Large fluctuations in blood bilirubin concentrations can also occur, even early in the disease, as a result of intermittent bile duct obstructions or bacterial cholangitis. Both albumin concentration and prothrombin time are normal in the disease's early stage. Later, when cirrhosis develops, albumin concentration falls and prothrombin time can be prolonged. The prothrombin time can also be prolonged prior to the development of cirrhosis secondary to decreased vitamin K absorption, in which case it will correct with the injection of vitamin K.

Immunological abnormalities are often, but not invariably, detectable in patients with PSC. None of them is specific to the diagnosis. About 30 percent of affected individuals have elevated blood gamma-globulin concentrations and about half have elevated total blood IgM concentrations. About 50 percent of patients have a particular type of autoantibody known (probably incorrectly) as *"antineutrophil cytoplasmic antibodies"* or *"ANCA."* These can also be detected in patients with inflammatory bowel disease without PSC. In PSC and inflammatory bowel disease, the ANCA are different than the classical ANCA found in patients with certain vasculitic diseases. Some patients with PSC may also have antismooth muscle or antinuclear antibodies.

Diagnosis of PSC is most reliably made by endoscopic retrograde cholangiopancreatography (ERCP). The findings include strictures and dilatations of the medium-sized and large bile ducts inside and outside the liver. The characteristic pattern is often described as "beads on a string" caused by the alternating widening and narrowing of the bile ducts. Liver biopsy in PSC is usually confirmatory, but rarely diagnostic. Sometimes, a very characteristic finding known as an "onion skin" lesion (layers of fibrosis tissue surrounding a bile duct) is seen on liver biopsy. Liver biopsy in PSC is also important in determining if the patient has cirrhosis.

Secondary causes of sclerosing cholangitis must be ruled out when making the diagnosis of PSC. Causes of secondary sclerosing cholangitis include drugs, bile duct cancers, and past biliary tree surgery. Infections of the bile ducts with cytomegalovirus (CMV) and *Crytosporidia* in patients with AIDS can also result in a picture similar to PSC. The causes of secondary sclerosing cholangitis can usually be eliminated based on patient history, physical examination, and appropriate laboratory tests.

Treatment and follow-up

Current medical therapy does not have a significant impact on PSC. Ursodiol (Actigall or Urso) improves laboratory test results but studies have demonstrated that it does not prolong survival until liver transplantation is necessary. Treatment in patients with PSC is directed at complications. Itching can be treated with bile acid-binding resins such as cholestyramine and, possibly, the opioid antagonist naltrexone. Deficiencies in fat-soluble vitamins, such as vitamin K and vitamin D, are treated by supplementation.

Episodes of bacterial cholangitis can be life threatening, and immediate antibiotic therapy in the hospital is necessary. There may be some role for dilatation of dominant bile duct strictures by ERCP in some cases of PSC, but there have been no controlled trials proving that this is effective. *If such a procedure is recommended, a physician with considerable experience in treating patients with PSC should be consulted.* Inappropriate or improperly performed procedures to dilate the bile ducts can be dangerous and lead to additional damage, worsening the patient's prognosis. As there is an increased incidence of cholangiocarcinoma in patients with PSC, this should always be suspected, especially in patients with long-standing disease whose condition worsens. Therefore, ERCP or CAT scan to look for bile duct cancer may be necessary in a patient whose condition deteriorates.

Liver transplantation is highly effective in the treatment of patients with advanced liver disease caused by PSC. Indications for liver transplantation are complications of cirrhosis. In some cases, patients with PSC and recurrent, life-threatening episodes of bacterial cholangitis warrant consideration for liver transplantation.

Inherited Liver Diseases

Some diseases result from alterations in a single gene. These diseases are generally referred to as "inherited" or "genetic." They are also said to demonstrate *Mendelian inheritance.* The term *Mendelian* derives from the monk Gregor Mendel, who was the first person to describe single gene inheritance based on his work breeding pea plants (an excellent database of human genetic disease is Dr. Victor McKusick's "Online Mendelian Inheritance in Man," which can be found on the World Wide Web at URL http://www3.ncbi.nlm.nih.gov/Omim/).

In genetic disorders, the normal gene is referred to as *wild-type* and the gene that causes the disease as *mutant.* In *autosomal dominant* disorders, affected individuals need possess only one mutant copy of the responsible gene to cause disease. In *autosomal recessive* disorders, an individual with the disease must have two copies of the mutant gene. Individuals with two copies of a mutant gene are said to be *homozygotes.* Individuals with one copy are *heterozygotes* or "carriers." Some genetic diseases are passed on by mutant genes on the X chromosome. In mammals, females have two X chromosomes and males only one. Therefore, in *X-linked* recessive disorders, men need have only one copy of a mutant gene to have a disease while women need to have two.

The most important inherited liver diseases are autosomal recessive. Therefore, a brief discussion on their pattern of inheritance is warranted. If a heterozygote, or "carrier," breeds with an individual with two wild-type genes, none of the offspring will have the disease but 50 percent of the offspring will be carriers of the mutant gene. If two carriers breed, 50 percent of the offspring will be carriers, with 25 percent having the disease and 25 percent having two copies of the wild-type gene. If an individual with the disease breeds with a carrier, 50 percent of the offspring will be carriers and 50 percent will have the disease. If two individuals with the disease breed, 100 percent of the offspring will have the disease. If someone with the disease breeds with a normal individual, all the offspring will be carriers. These situations are outlined schematically in Figure 4.6.

A detailed discussion of all inherited diseases that affect the liver is beyond the scope of this book. This chapter will address the "big three": hereditary hemochromatosis, alpha-1-antitrypsin deficiency, and Wilson disease. A discussion of Gilbert syndrome, a very common inherited condition that causes elevated unconjugated bilirubin concentrations in the blood and sometimes jaundice, is also included. For additional details on these conditions, and for information on the more esoteric genetic liver diseases not discussed in this book, I refer all readers to "Online Mendelian Inheritance in Man" (http://www3.ncbi. nlm.nih.gov/Omim/) on the Internet.

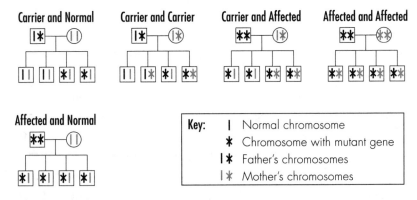

Figure 4.6. *Schematic diagram showing patterns of inheritance in an autosomal recessive genetic disease.*

Hemochromatosis

Hereditary hemochromatosis, or primary hemochromatosis, is the most common inherited disease in persons of European descent. It occurs in 3 to 5 people in 1,000. About 1 in 10 individuals are carriers who possess one copy of the mutant gene. People with hereditary hemochromatosis have increased absorption of iron resulting in excess deposition in the liver, heart, joints, and other organs. This abnormal accumulation of iron can cause cirrhosis, heart disease, arthritis, diabetes mellitus, pituitary gland abnormalities, and a bronze coloring of the skin.

The problem with hemochromatosis is that in most cases, the disease is not diagnosed until complications develop. Most individuals will have high body iron for many years without symptoms. Men usually present with symptoms earlier in life than women because younger women constantly lose iron during menstruation. Many patients have cirrhosis of unclear cause until a liver biopsy indicates increased iron content. Sometimes, patients will present with complications from iron deposition in other organs such as arthritis, diabetes, or heart disease. These may occur along with, or independently from, liver disease.

The diagnosis of hereditary hemochromatosis is *suspected* from the results of blood tests suggesting elevated body iron concentrations. There are three simple blood tests related to iron metabolism: iron, transferrin saturation, and ferritin. Elevations in these, especially elevations in both transferrin saturation and ferritin together, suggest, but are not specific for, hemochromatosis. A diagnosis of hereditary hemochromatosis is usually made by liver biopsy and determination of liver iron content. The doctor should send a sample of liver tissue obtained from the biopsy for measurement of iron content. In hereditary hemochromatosis, the liver iron content is significantly elevated.

For many years, it was known that the gene responsible for hereditary hemochromatosis was on chromosome 6. In 1996, investigators at the biotechnology company Mercator Genetics identified a candidate gene for hemochromatosis on this chromosome. They initially called this gene HLA-H, but the name HFE is now recommended for this gene. It appears that about 90 percent of individuals with hereditary hemochromatosis have the same mutation in the HFE gene, which can be detected in the laboratory.

The genetic test for mutations in the HFE gene now plays an important role in diagnosis of carriers and patients with hereditary hemochromatosis. It is especially important in screening the children, brothers, and sisters of patients with the disease as they are also at risk. Some doctors may argue that liver biopsy is not essential if hereditary hemochromatosis is diagnosed by genetic testing. Others will state that biopsy is still necessary to establish the extent of liver disease and the presence or absence of cirrhosis. Because the genetic test is relatively new, no studies have yet been completed assessing the need for liver biopsies in patients in whom hereditary hemochromatosis is diagnosed using the genetic test.

There is an effective treatment for hereditary hemochromatosis if the disease is diagnosed early. As the damage to organs in hemochromatosis results from excessive iron deposition, lowering the body's total iron load will prevent it. The treatment, therefore, is "blood letting" or, in medical terminology, phlebotomy. Repeated phlebotomy is performed to reduce the red blood cell count to a level slightly below normal. It is maintained there by periodic repeat phlebotomies. If hereditary hemochromatosis is diagnosed early, phlebotomy is extremely effective in preventing ensuing complications. Unfortunately, hereditary hemochromatosis is frequently not diagnosed until it is rather late and organ damage, such as cirrhosis, has already occurred.

Secondary hemochromatosis is a condition that mimics hereditary hemochromatosis. Secondary hemochromatosis results from iron deposition in the body, including the liver, secondary to nongenetic causes. A common cause is repeated blood transfusions over many years, as may be necessary in individuals with blood diseases such as thalassemias. Some individuals with alcoholic liver disease also develop secondary hemochromatosis for unclear reasons.

Alpha-1-Antitrypsin Deficiency

Inherited deficiency of the protein alpha-1-antitrypsin, which is synthesized in the liver and secreted into the blood, can cause lung and liver disease. The major function of alpha-1-antitrypsin in the body is to inhibit the function of an enzyme known as elastase. Elastase breaks down a structural component of the lungs known as elastin. If its activity is not partially inhibited by alpha-1-antitrypsin in the body, excessive lung damage and emphysema may occur.

Certain mutations in the gene for alpha-1-antitrypsin lead to production of an abnormal form that is not properly secreted from liver cells. The mutant form of alpha-1-antitrypsin that causes this abnormality is known as the Z mutation. In individuals who have inherited two abnormal Z genes, about 85 percent of synthesized alpha-1-antitrypsin accumulates in hepatocytes and forms aggregates. Retained aggregates of the Z form of alpha-1-antitrypsin in the liver can cause hepatitis and eventually cirrhosis.

Between 12 and 15 percent of individuals who have inherited two abnormal alpha-1-antitrypsin Z genes develop liver disease. About 10 percent develop cirrhosis in early infancy or early childhood. The remainder are first diagnosed with chronic liver disease as adults. Patients with the Z form mutation are generally not at increased risk for lung disease because the little bit of alpha-1-antitrypsin that makes it into their blood inhibits elastase. On the other hand, people with other mutant forms of alpha-1-antitrypsin get lung disease because either an inactive form is secreted from the liver or none is made at all. These people, however, do not get liver disease because these other mutant forms do not accumulate in the liver.

The diagnosis of alpha-1-antitrypsin deficiency is made by measuring the amount of alpha-1-antitrypsin in the blood. Patients with two abnormal Z genes have blood concentrations about 85 percent normal. To distinguish the Z mutation from other mutations with decreased amounts of blood alpha-1-antitrypsin, a genetic test is available to directly detect the mutation in the alpha-1-antitrypsin gene. This test can be used to diagnose the condition prenatally if a mother is at risk for passing on the disease to her baby. Abnormal accumulation of alpha-1-antitrypsin can also be observed on liver biopsy in patients with two abnormal Z genes.

Liver transplantation is the only means of treatment for liver disease caused by alpha-1-antitrypsin deficiency. Transplantation is performed when complications of cirrhosis develop.

Wilson Disease

Wilson disease is an inherited disorder that primarily affects the brain and liver. Patients suffer from neurological, psychiatric, blood, and/or liver problems. The Wilson disease gene encodes a protein that most likely transports copper in or out of cells. In individuals with two mutant forms of this gene, copper accumulates in the liver, brain, and other organs. There is decreased secretion of copper into the bile and increased excretion of copper in the urine. About 85 percent of patients with Wilson disease also have low levels of ceruloplasmin, a copper binding protein that circulates in the blood.

The age of onset of symptoms in patients with Wilson disease varies considerably. About 50 percent of patients develop symptoms by age fifteen. Almost all have symptoms by the time they are age forty. Very rarely, patients with Wilson disease may not have symptoms until they are in their fifties. About half of patients first present to medical attention because of liver disease, about one-third with neurological symptoms, about 15 percent with blood problems, and 10 percent with psychiatric abnormalities.

Neurological symptoms usually appear in adolescents and young adults. At first, they are very subtle. A common initial presentation is deteriorating performance in school not related to an intellectual deficiency. More obvious symptoms include lack of coordination, tremors, clumsiness, and difficulty walking. Wilson disease can also lead to the development of debilitating nerve and muscle abnormalities and seizures. Psychiatric abnormalities predominate in some patients and include psychosis, manic-depression, aggressive behaviors, and dementia. These are usually diagnosed in teenagers who may be hospitalized in psychiatric institutions before the diagnosis of Wilson disease is made.

About 15 percent of patients with Wilson disease present with blood abnormalities. The blood disorder in Wilson disease is intravascular hemolysis, which is destruction of red blood cells within the bloodstream. Hemolysis is usually of sudden onset and can be very serious and even life threatening. More often, it is transient and resolves spontaneously.

Liver involvement in Wilson disease can mimic many other disorders. Patients can present with signs and symptoms of chronic or acute hepatitis. Some present with clinical symptoms resembling fulminant hepatic failure. Others first present with cirrhosis. Most common are patients with Wilson disease whose illness resembles chronic hepatitis that progresses to cirrhosis over several years.

Wilson disease should be suspected in all young individuals who present with liver disease, especially if there is a family history of liver disease, neurological, or psychiatric disorders. Several tests are used to establish the diagnosis. Most patients have a characteristic physical sign known as a Kayser-Fleischer ring. These are brownish discolorations of the part of the cornea (surface of the eye) surrounding the iris (the part of the eye that is colored). They probably result from abnormal copper deposition. They can be identified by an optometrist or ophthalmologist using a slit-lamp. Kayser-Fleischer rings are almost always present in patients with both Wilson disease and neurological symptoms, but may not be present in patients suffering from liver disease only.

In blood tests, the diagnosis of Wilson disease is suspected due to low ceruloplasmin concentration, which is found in about 85 percent of individuals with the disease. A low blood ceruloplasmin concentration in a person with Kayser-Fleischer rings essentially confirms the diagnosis of Wilson disease. The amount of copper in a twenty-four-hour urine sample is also elevated in patients with Wilson disease. It may also be elevated in individuals with cirrhosis from other causes. All untreated patients having Wilson disease exhibit significantly elevated concentrations of liver copper; however, this may also be observed in patients with other forms of liver disease. Nonetheless, measurement of liver copper content in tissue obtained at liver biopsy is an important test to establish the diagnosis. Liver biopsy, of course, will also establish the extent of liver damage.

Genetic tests for Wilson disease are available in research laboratories. Because many different mutations in the Wilson disease gene can cause the condition, the entire gene may have to be sequenced (unless the specific mutation in a family member is known). This makes genetic testing laborious at the present time. If the particular mutation in an individual is known, genetic testing of family members becomes somewhat easier.

D-penicillamine is an effective treatment for Wilson disease. It binds to copper and helps removes it from the body. Treatment can reverse neurological and psychiatric symptoms and some aspects of liver disease. Cirrhosis, of course, is not reversible, so effective treatment is aided by early diagnosis. If the diagnosis is made in an asymptomatic person, for example, a family member of someone with Wilson disease, all complications and symptoms can be prevented if the individual continues on therapy with D-penicillamine. In patients with both Wilson disease and end-stage cirrhosis, liver transplantation may be necessary. It may also be effective in sudden onset liver failure caused by Wilson disease.

Congenital Disorders of Bilirubin Metabolism

Several inherited diseases affect the metabolism of bilirubin in the liver. Most are very rare abnormalities resulting from either the defective conjugation of bilirubin or the abnormal secretion of conjugated bilirubin into the bile. The first type causes elevations in unconjugated bilirubin and the second type causes elevations in conjugated bilirubin in the blood. These disorders usually present as jaundice at birth. A detailed discussion of each is beyond the scope of this book, but some of the better known of these "classical" inherited liver diseases are explained briefly in Table 4.12.

Gilbert Syndrome

One very common inherited disorder of bilirubin metabolism, usually diagnosed in adults, is Gilbert syndrome. Gilbert syndrome is *not* a serious condition but is often of concern to patients. In addition, it sometimes leads to extensive and inappropriate testing by doctors. In fact, Gilbert syndrome is not a "disease" but a normal variant in which patients have mildly elevated unconjugated bilirubin concentrations in their blood. They may also occasionally be jaundiced. These abnormalities are of no real clinical significance. Gilbert syndrome tends to run in families but does not always demonstrate strict Mendelian inheritance patterns.

Gilbert syndrome is probably caused by mildly decreased activity of the enzyme UDP-glucuronosyltransferase that catalyzes the conjugation of bilirubin in the liver. Subtle mutations in the regulatory region of the gene encoding this enzyme have been described. There may be other causes of Gilbert syndrome, such as decreased uptake of unconjugated bilirubin from the blood by hepatocytes. As a result of these abnormalities, the concentration of unconjugated bilirubin in the blood is abnormally elevated.

Gilbert syndrome is most frequently discovered when someone is found to have a slightly elevated total bilirubin concentration on blood tests taken for other reasons. The blood bilirubin concentration is usually less than 2 mg per deciliter and the individual is not jaundiced. The indirect (unconjugated) bilirubin

Table 4.12. *Rare inherited disorders of bilirubin metabolism that cause jaundice.*

Disorders of impaired conjugation of bilirubin

Crigler-Najjar syndrome type 1—Results from absent activity of the enzyme that conjugates bilirubin to its glucuronide form. Inherited in an autosomal recessive manner. May be fatal in childhood without liver transplantation.

Crigler-Najjar syndrome type 2—Results from decreased activity of the enzyme that conjugates bilirubin to its glucuronide form. Autosomal recessive inheritance. Serum bilirubin concentrations usually range from 8 to 20 mg/dl. Patients generally do well except for being jaundiced.

Disorders of impaired secretion of bilirubin

Dubin-Johnson syndrome—Results from mutations in a protein that transports conjugated bilirubin out of hepatocytes and into the bile. Inherited in an autosomal recessive manner. Very rare except in Persian Jews where it is seen in 1 in 1,300 individuals. A dark pigment found in hepatocytes. Generally benign course.

Rotor syndrome—Autosomal recessive inheritance. Very rare. Cause not clear. Benign course.

concentration in the blood is elevated but the conjugated (direct) bilirubin concentration is normal. Some people with Gilbert syndrome, however, may actually present to doctors because of jaundice, especially while suffering from an unrelated illness. This is because the condition is exacerbated by fasting, stress, and infections. In such instances, the blood bilirubin concentration may reach 6 mg per deciliter.

A diagnosis of Gilbert syndrome is made by finding the characteristic elevation of the blood indirect bilirubin concentration with a normal direct bilirubin concentration in blood tests. However, similar laboratory test results can be seen in disorders in which bilirubin production is increased, such as those causing abnormal breakdown of red blood cells. Therefore, these should be excluded as a cause of the laboratory abnormality. Few, if any, acquired liver diseases in *adults* cause elevations of the indirect bilirubin with a normal direct bilirubin. This means that other blood tests related to the liver such as the aminotransferase and alkaline phosphatase activities, should be normal. (However, Gilbert syndrome can occur in individuals with other liver diseases.) A diagnosis of Gilbert syndrome is further supported by an elevated blood indirect bilirubin concentration in a relative. If the diagnosis remains in question, the drug phenobarbital can be given and the blood bilirubin concentration measured again, as phenobarbital will decrease bilirubin concentration in an individual with Gilbert syndrome.

An extensive search for structural liver disease is *not* necessary in individuals with Gilbert syndrome. Unfortunately, some doctors embark on costly and unnecessary evaluations. They sometimes even order CAT scans and ultrasound scans that are not indicated, as liver diseases detectable on these studies would cause elevations in the *direct* blood bilirubin concentration.

Individuals with Gilbert syndrome have normal life spans. They do not suffer from a disease. No treatment is indicated.

Liver Cancers, Tumors, Cysts, and Abscesses

There are many different abnormal masses that can be present in the liver. These are most frequently discovered first as "lesions" on radiological tests such as ultrasound or CAT scans. Sometimes, these scans are ordered to evaluate patients with clinical signs of liver disease or due to blood test results that suggest liver problems. In other instances, lesions are found in the liver on radiological scans performed for other purposes, for example, an ultrasound examination done during pregnancy, or to examine the gallbladder or kidneys.

Many people ask me about "lesions on the liver" (some ask about "spots on the liver") as if it is a specific disease. The term *lesion* (and *spot*) is a nonspecific, general term that refers to any abnormality seen on any radiological test. Radiological studies are definitive enough to diagnose only a few "lesions" seen in the liver. In most cases, radiological scans alone are *not* sufficient to determine what they are, and tissue sampling, that is, biopsy, is necessary to make a diagnosis. In this section, I will review briefly some important points about cancers, other tumors, cysts, and abscesses that can be found in the liver.

Cancer

The term *liver cancer* really does not refer to a particular diagnosis. The reason is that many different cancers can affect the liver. Most "liver cancers" that people in the Western world refer to are cancers that originate in other organs and spread to the liver via the bloodstream. In the East, most liver cancers are just that, being hepatocellular carcinomas that originate in the liver itself. This is a very important distinction.

Metastatic cancer

Metastatic cancers are tumors that spread from the organ of origin to other nearby or distant sites. Because of its rich blood supply, the liver is a common site where cancer will spread. Malignant tumors arising in virtually any organ can spread to the liver. Some of the most common cancers that metastasize to the liver are those originating in the colon, pancreas, lung, and breast. These cancers are known as *carcinomas* because they arise in epithelial tissues. Lymphomas and leukemias, cancers that originate in the lymph nodes and bone marrow, respectively, can also invade the liver. So can sarcomas, which are cancers that originate in tissues such as muscle or cartilage.

Once a diagnosis of cancer metastatic to the liver is made, and the tissue of origin determined (usually requiring a biopsy at a specific site), treatment of metastatic liver cancer usually falls into the domain of an *oncologist*—a medical cancer specialist. Several different types of treatment may be offered. In some cases, procedures can be performed that relieve symptoms and, perhaps, prolong life. They are usually not curative. Chemotherapy can be instilled directly into the liver via an implanted pump. Surgeons can resect one or two isolated, metastatic tumors. Large metastatic tumors can be treated by embolysis. In this procedure, a catheter is passed through the hepatic artery to vessels feeding the tumor, and drugs or other materials are injected to clot off the tumor's blood supply. Many experimental therapies for metastatic cancers are also under investigation in clinical trials at numerous medical schools and hospitals. Organizations such as the American Cancer Society (http://www.cancer.org) and the National Cancer Institute (http://www.nci.nih.gov) can provide information for patients and doctors interested in such trials.

Most patients with cancers that have metastasized to the liver have a very poor prognosis. Once a carcinoma has spread to the liver, the patient's life expectancy is usually a couple of years at most. A notable exception is testicular cancer, which is very responsive to chemotherapy and can be cured. Some types of lymphomas and leukemias that involve the liver may also respond very well to chemotherapy and can be cured.

Primary Liver Cancer

There are two types of primary liver cancer; both cancers originate in the liver itself. *Hepatocellular carcinoma* is cancer that arises from hepatocytes. Intrahepatic *cholangiocarcinoma* is cancer that arises from bile duct cells within the liver. (Technically, these cancers may arise from "liver stem cells" that are normally destined to become either hepatocytes or bile ducts; this point has not been resolved.)

Hepatocellular carcinoma, although relatively rare in the U.S., is either the number one or number two cause of cancer death worldwide (along with lung cancer). About 80 percent of people with hepatocellular carcinomas have cirrhosis. This type of cancer is especially common in parts of Asia and Africa where hepatitis B virus infection, which is a major risk factor, is endemic. Chronic hepatitis C virus infection is probably the next leading cause. As discussed in earlier sections of this book, patients chronically infected with hepatitis B virus and hepatitis C virus should probably have some type of periodic "screening" for hepatocellular carcinoma. Hepatocellular carcinoma may also develop in patients with cirrhosis from any cause (except, according to some investigators, Wilson disease). Aflatoxins have also been implicated as a major risk factor for causing hepatocellular carcinoma. Although virtually nonexistent in the U.S., aflatoxins, which are produced by a mold that is a contaminant of nuts (most commonly peanuts), grains, and beans, are common in other parts of the world. They are commonly present in food in some parts of the world where hepatitis B virus infection is endemic.

Hepatocellular carcinomas are usually discovered as masses on CAT scans or ultrasound scans. The majority of patients with hepatocellular carcinomas have cirrhosis. In patients who have cirrhosis, a sudden deterioration in clinical condition may provide a clue to the presence of a hepatocellular carcinoma. Sometimes they will cause pain. Rising blood alkaline phosphatase activity may also suggest the diagnosis. *Alpha-fetoprotein* is a useful marker for diagnosis of hepatocellular carcinoma. It is often measured as part of routine "screening" in patients with chronic hepatitis B and chronic hepatitis C. Rising blood alpha-fetoprotein concentration in someone with chronic liver disease suggests the development of hepatocellular carcinoma. CAT or ultrasound scans should be performed in such instances. About 70 percent of patients with hepatocellular carcinoma have elevated blood alpha-fetoprotein concentrations. It is not specific for hepatocellular carcinoma as individuals with other types of cancer—especially testicular—may also have elevated blood concentrations.

The definitive diagnosis of hepatocellular carcinoma is made by biopsy. Usually, the liver mass is biopsied by a radiologist under CAT scan or ultrasound guidance. Sometimes, it is biopsied using a laparoscope, a fiber-optic instrument that is inserted into the abdomen. Occasionally, open surgical biopsy is necessary.

Hepatocellular carcinoma is curable by surgery only if the tumor is small. Surgery may not be possible in individuals with advanced cirrhosis. If surgery is contemplated, extensive presurgical evaluation by CAT scanning, magnetic resonance scanning, and angiography (injection of dye into the hepatic artery followed by X-ray) is required. Some patients with cirrhosis and small hepatocellular carcinomas confined to the liver may be treated by liver transplantation. For large tumors, or cancer that has spread beyond the liver, chemotherapy, ligating (tying) or embolization (clotting) of the hepatic artery, alcohol injection into the tumor, or radiation may relieve symptoms and prolong life, though none is curative. Patients may also opt for enrollment in clinical trials utilizing these and other experimental procedures.

The prognosis after treatment of hepatocellular carcinoma depends upon the size of the tumor and the extent to which the liver has already damaged been by cirrhosis. For patients with hepatocellular carcinomas that are deemed to be surgically resectable, the five-year survival rate after surgery is 10 to 30 percent. Rare hepatocellular carcinomas, often discovered in young women without cirrhosis, are a fibrolamellar variant that has a better prognosis after surgical resection. Patients with advanced cirrhosis generally do poorly after surgical resection, and should be considered for possible liver transplantation if the tumors are small and have not spread. At the present time, not much data are available regarding survival rates after liver transplantation for small tumors. For patients with hepatocellular carcinomas confined to the liver, in whom complete surgical removal of the tumor is not possible, the five-year survival rate is about 1 percent. Virtually no patients with hepatocellular carcinoma that has spread beyond the liver survive for long, and most die within a few months.

Cholangiocarcinomas can arise in both the liver and the bile ducts outside the liver. Cholangiocarcinomas are usually discovered first on radiological studies and diagnosed by biopsy. *Carcinoembryonal antigen,* also known as CEA, may be elevated in the blood of patients with this tumor. In some parts of the world, liver fluke *(Clonorchis sinensis)* infection is a predisposing risk for development of cholangiocarcinoma. Patients with primary sclerosing cholangitis are also at increased risk for development of cholangiocarcinomas.

The prognosis of cholangiocarcinoma is similar to that for hepatocellular carcinoma. Small tumors may be surgically resected in rare cases only; otherwise, the patient may undergo liver transplantation. Patients with cholangiocarcinomas that cannot be surgically resected, or have spread beyond the liver, have a poor prognosis.

Hemangioma

Hemangioma (more precisely, cavernous hemangioma) is the most common benign liver tumor found in adults. They are more commonly found in older persons and rarely identified in young children. For reasons that are unclear, hemangiomas are more common in women, and estrogen may increase their size. Hemangiomas are composed of vascular channels that may contain clotted blood and fibrous tissue. They can range in size and be as large as several inches across.

Patients with hemangiomas are usually asymptomatic and the condition is almost always diagnosed incidentally when ultrasound, CAT scan, or other imaging studies are undertaken for other reasons. In some instances, a patient with a hemangioma will present with abdominal pain, nausea, vomiting, or a mass that can be felt in the upper abdomen. Very rarely, patients will present with anemia or low platelet counts resulting from red blood cells or platelets that are trapped and/or destroyed within the tumor. In very rare instances, a hemangioma can rupture, usually after abdominal trauma.

A diagnosis of hemangioma is made using special imaging studies. Routine ultrasound may be suggestive but usually is not diagnostic. Definitive diagnosis can usually be made by a tagged red blood cell scan, MRI scan, or dynamic CAT scan performed after intravenous contrast dye is given.

Cavernous hemangioma causes much more worry and concern for patients than actual problems. Complications are extremely rare and, in virtually all cases, nothing has to be done once a diagnosis is made. If a patient with a liver hemangioma exhibits none or only minimal symptoms, no treatment is necessary. *In very rare cases,* symptomatic hemangiomas may be treated by surgical resection.

Hemangioendothelioma is a rare tumor occurring only in infants and young children. It is sometimes associated with heart failure. Children with this type of hemangioma may die as a result of heart failure or rupture. If they survive, the tumor usually disappears as they grow.

Benign nodular lesions

Several nodular tumor-like lesions can affect the liver. They are often first suspected based on radiological scans with a biopsy required for definitive diagnosis. All of these conditions are rather rare.

Adenomas are benign tumors that rarely occur in the liver. Liver adenomas are much more common in women and it is possible, but not conclusively proven, that they may be associated with long-term use of birth control pills. In many cases, they are first identified through radiological studies conducted for other indications. Sometimes patients present with a mass or pain in the right upper abdomen. If an adenoma is suspected, biopsy is usually done surgically because the tumor has a rich blood supply and needle biopsy can be dangerous. Because adenomas can rupture, surgical treatment is often recommend.

Focal nodular hyperplasia is characterized by benign nodules in the liver. Like hepatic adenomas, focal nodular hyperplasia occurs primarily in women. Birth control pills may predispose women to this condition. Most patients with focal nodular hyperplasia do not have symptoms but, sometimes, a mass can be felt in the abdomen. Small lesions may have to be resected because of the chance of rupture.

Nodular regenerative hyperplasia is a condition characterized by nodules without scar tissue throughout the liver. Patients with nodular regenerative hyperplasia can sometimes develop portal hypertension and associated complications.

Partial nodular transformation is characterized by nodules surrounded by scar tissue in the liver. Patients with partial nodular transformation usually have portal hypertension.

Other liver tumors

Many different rare tumors can involve the liver. Most are benign and do not require treatment. They are usually discovered by radiological scanning, sometimes in patients who complain of abdominal pain or other symptoms suggesting a liver mass. Diagnosis usually involves biopsy.

Cysts

Cysts are cell-lined structures filled with fluid that occur within tissues. Many different types of cysts affect the liver. Most are benign and of little consequence. They are usually diagnosed by their characteristic appearance on radiological procedures. Some liver cysts can be quite large. Some inherited diseases, for example, Caroli disease, cause multiple cysts in the kidney and liver. In some forms of inherited polycystic kidney disease, liver cysts can also be seen. Very rarely, cystic lesions can be malignant. Whether or not a cyst needs to be worked up further after its discovery on a radiological test depends upon the radiological appearance and other factors. They usually do not require further investigation.

An infectious disease that can cause cysts in the liver is echinococcosis or hydatid cyst disease. It is caused by small tapeworms of the genus *Echinococcus* that usually live in the intestines of dogs and other animals. Echinococcus is transmitted to humans by contact with animal feces. The disease is rare in the U.S. and is most common in sheep and cattle raising areas. Hydatid cysts are treated by surgery and/or the drug mebendazole.

Abscesses

Abscesses are walled-off areas of infection filled with pus. They can occur in the liver. Liver abscesses caused by bacteria usually occur after surgery, injury, or as a result of blood infection. Liver abscesses can also be caused by parasites, including infection with amoeba *(Entamoeba histolycia)*. Patients with liver abscesses usually have signs and symptoms of infection, such as fever and chills. They may have pain in the right upper quadrant of the abdomen. Abscesses are treated with appropriate antibiotics. Surgical drainage may also be necessary.

Budd-Chiari Syndrome

Budd-Chiari syndrome is thrombosis (clotting) of the hepatic vein. It can present as an acute or chronic illness. Most patients are ill for less than six months before seeking medical attention. The most common symptom in Budd-Chiari syndrome is ascites, which occurs in 70 to 90 percent of patients. Patients can also have abnormal blood tests that indicate liver disease. Some individuals with Budd-Chiari syndrome may be jaundiced.

Most patients with Budd-Chiari syndrome have an underlying condition that predisposes to blood clotting. About 10 percent have *polycythemia vera,* a condition in which abnormal amounts of red blood cells are produced, making the blood more likely to clot because it is too thick. Some cancers can also cause enhanced blood clotting. About 10 percent of patients with Budd-Chiari syndrome take birth control pills, which also may predispose them to blood clotting. It is not clear if these individuals also have blood clotting disorders that have not been diagnosed. Patients who suffer from Budd-Chiari syndrome without apparent predisposing conditions may also have blood clotting disorders that have not been, or cannot yet be, diagnosed.

In a patient with Budd-Chiari syndrome, the examining doctors often first suspect cirrhosis as the primary cause of the symptoms. Budd-Chiari syndrome is then diagnosed based on characteristic findings on liver biopsy. Various radiological tests, such as ultrasound scan with Doppler studies, may also suggest the diagnosis. Direct catheterization of the hepatic vein with injection of dye followed by X-ray is the definitive test to indicate that it is clotted.

Patients with Budd-Chiari syndrome who have deteriorating liver function and/or complications of portal hypertension usually need to be treated by liver transplantation. Other surgical procedures have been used with varying degrees of success. In some cases, however, the underlying condition that caused the hepatic vein thrombosis excludes transplantation as a treatment option.

Congestive Heart Failure

In congestive heart failure, the heart fails to pump blood effectively. As a result, blood backs up in other tissues and organs, including the liver. Figure 4.7 shows how heart pump failure leads to congestion of blood in the liver. Chronic congestion of blood in the liver can lead to fibrosis and cirrhosis. This condition is often referred to as "cardiac cirrhosis."

The treatment approach for a patient with congestive heart failure is to treat the heart disease to prevent the cirrhosis from developing further. Congestive heart failure and constrictive pericarditis (inflammation of the lining around the heart leading to abnormal pumping) can cause ascites and edema prior to causing cirrhosis. On first impression, if poor heart function is

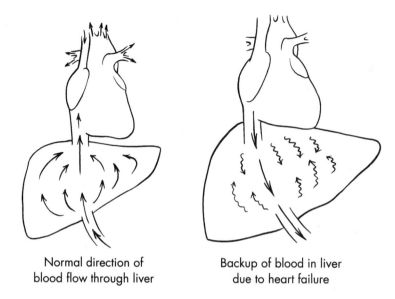

Normal direction of
blood flow through liver

Backup of blood in liver
due to heart failure

Figure 4.7. *Schematic diagram showing how congestive heart failure causes congestion of blood in the liver.*

Congestion of blood in the liver for long periods of time can lead to cirrhosis.

Illustration by Elizabeth Weadon Massari

not obvious, patients with congestive heart failure may be misdiagnosed as suffering from cirrhosis.

Shock Liver

Shock liver, or ischemic hepatitis, is caused by lack of oxygen delivery (ischemia) to liver cells. Causes of shock liver include heart failure, heatstroke, overwhelming infection (sepsis), burns, dehydration, and hemorrhage. In most cases, shock liver is accompanied by acute renal failure that similarly results from lack of blood flow and oxygen delivery to the kidneys. Although often present, low blood pressure (hypotension) is not present in all cases of shock liver.

In shock liver, numerous hepatocytes suddenly die and intracellular contents leak into the blood. As a result, blood ALT and AST activities are usually massively elevated. The peak elevations in blood ALT and AST activities occur within two days after ischemic injury. This is followed by a return of the markedly abnormal laboratory values to normal or near-normal within seven to ten days.

Shock liver can cause fulminant hepatic failure. Treatment is directed at the underlying cause, for example, treating infection with antibiotics or treating hemorrhage with intravenous fluids and blood transfusions. Patients with shock liver die either from the underlying problem or from fulminant hepatic failure, or gradually recover if the underlying condition is reversible. Emergency liver transplantation can be performed in cases of fulminant hepatic failure where the underlying cause of shock liver is reversed.

Gallbladder and Bile Ducts

The smallest bile ducts within the liver merge into successively larger and larger ducts until they form the common hepatic duct that emerges from the liver. The common hepatic duct merges with the cystic duct, which is connected to the gallbladder, to form the common bile duct. The common bile duct then empties into the small intestine. The pancreatic duct, which drains the pancreas, also usually merges with the common bile duct at about the place where it empties into the small intestine. The anatomy of the gallbladder and bile ducts is shown in Figure 4.8.

Disorders that affect the bile ducts and gallbladder may cause liver disease. Most importantly, bile duct obstruction resulting from gallstones, tumors, or improperly performed surgery can cause liver disease. In addition, disorders of the pancreas such as pancreatitis (pancreas inflammation) can also cause liver problems.

Acute total bile duct obstruction usually causes sudden onset jaundice. For example, a common presentation of pancreatic

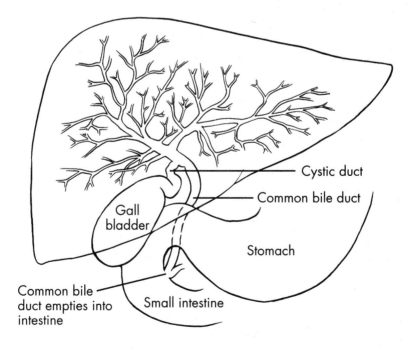

Figure 4.8. *Anatomy of the gallbladder and bile ducts.*
Illustration by Elizabeth Weadon Massari

cancer is jaundice because the tumor blocks the common bile duct. Complete obstruction of the common bile duct by a gallstone can cause sudden onset pain, fever, and jaundice. The blood alkaline phosphatase and GGTP activities will be elevated. Partial obstruction may not cause jaundice but will cause elevations in blood alkaline phosphatase and GGTP activities. Bile duct obstructions can lead to bacterial infections of the bile ducts *(cholangitis)* that can ascend into the liver *(ascending cholangitis)*.

Long-standing obstruction of the external bile ducts will lead to biliary cirrhosis. Throughout the underdeveloped world, chronic complications of gallbladder surgery are a common cause of cirrhosis. Fortunately, this is very rare in the U.S. and other countries where high-quality medical care is available.

The treatment of liver complications due to bile duct obstruction is to treat the bile duct, gallbladder, or pancreatic problem causing it. This usually involves opening an obstruction or treating an infection. Obstructions can be corrected surgically, or more and more commonly by endoscopic procedures. ERCP can be modified to extract stones from the common bile duct or place stents through obstructing tumors. If recurrent gallstones is a problem, the gallbladder can be removed.

Liver Diseases of Infants and Young Children

Children can suffer from many of the same liver diseases as adults. There are some liver diseases unique to children that do not affect adults, however; kernicterus, or bilirubin toxicity, occurs in infants only.

Kernicterus

At very high blood concentrations, unconjugated bilirubin is toxic to the brain. Bilirubin toxicity is known as *kernicterus.* Kernicterus occurs in newborn babies with very high unconjugated bilirubin concentrations, usually above 20 mg per deciliter of blood. In newborn babies, the unconjugated bilirubin can readily cross the undeveloped blood-brain barrier. In addition, the brain of a newborn is very sensitive to the toxic accumulation of bilirubin.

Kernicterus can occur in infants with genetic disorders of bilirubin metabolism (see Table 4.12). It can also occur in very premature babies, and some mature babies with neonatal jaundice (see below). The encephalopathy of kernicterus usually manifests as refusal to feed, high-pitched crying, and increased muscle tone. If severe, the baby can die. Babies who survive often have irreversible problems including mental retardation, deafness, and cerebral palsy.

Infants with highly elevated unconjugated blood bilirubin concentrations may be treated by phototherapy to prevent kernicterus. In phototherapy, the infant is placed under visible light that sometimes is greenish. Light induces subtle changes in the orientation of atoms around certain chemical bonds in the unconjugated bilirubin molecule. As a result, bilirubin becomes increasingly water soluble and is excreted in the kidneys. These more soluble forms of bilirubin are referred to as "photoisomers."

Neonatal Jaundice

Many infants are born with mild elevations in their blood unconjugated bilirubin concentrations. In most cases, this is due to the condition neonatal jaundice or neonatal hyperbilirubine-mia. Neonatal jaundice occurs because enzymes and other cellular factors involved in bilirubin metabolism in the liver are not yet mature. The activity of UDP-glucuronosyltransferase, the enzyme that conjugates bilirubin, is decreased in newborn babies, especially those born premature. In addition, newborns usually have increased destruction of red blood cells leading to increased production of bilirubin.

In most cases, there are no untoward consequences of neonatal jaundice. The condition usually resolves soon after birth. Infants with neonatal jaundice, usually those born premature, are at risk for kernicterus if the blood unconjugated bilirubin concentrations are very high. These babies may be treated with phototherapy until they mature to the point when their own livers can adequately conjugate bilirubin and secrete it into bile.

Biliary Atresia

Biliary atresia is defined as the lack of a lumen in part or all of the bile ducts outside of the liver, causing complete obstruction of bile flow. In reality, there may be some bile flow, but it is severely decreased. Newborn babies with biliary atresia present with jaundice, and the challenge for the pediatrician is to differentiate this condition from other, less serious causes of jaundice.

Biliary atresia occurs in about 1 in 10,000 to 15,000 live births. In some cases, it is associated with other congenital malformations. *Alagille syndrome* is an inherited condition characterized by biliary atresia and decreased numbers of smaller bile ducts within the liver. Children with Alagille syndrome suffer from associated conditions that include abnormal pigmentation in the eyes, heart valve problems, bone problems, and neurological changes. They also have characteristic physical features such as broad forehead, pointed jaw, and bulbous tip of the nose. There are also cases of biliary atresia with decreased bile ducts in the liver without these syndromatic malformations.

Without treatment, the prognosis of babies with biliary atresia is extremely poor. Most die within one year of diagnosis. Some surgical procedures have been shown to prolong survival, such as the commonly performed Kasai procedure. These surgical procedures attempt to restore the flow of bile from the liver to the intestine. They are usually of temporary benefit and, in the long term, most children do not do well. Liver transplantation provides the best overall option for children with biliary atresia, even for those who have had previous Kasai operations. Liver transplantation not only reestablishes bile flow but also replaces an organ that may be damaged as a result of bile duct obstruction. The long-term prognosis for most children who receive liver transplantation for biliary atresia is excellent.

Hepatoblastoma

Hepatoblastoma is a malignant primary liver cancer that essentially occurs only in children, usually within the first three years of life. Small, isolated tumors may be cured by surgical resection. Babies with large hepatoblastomas, or ones that have spread beyond the liver, have a very poor prognosis.

Liver Diseases and Pregnancy

Pregnant women can also suffer from the same liver disease as other adults. The most common liver disease that occurs during pregnancy is, in fact, viral hepatitis. However, there are several liver diseases unique to pregnancy:

- Liver involvement in hyperemesis gravidum (morning sickness)
- Cholestasis of pregnancy
- Fatty liver of pregnancy
- Liver involvement in eclampsia and pre-eclampsia
- HELLP syndrome

Liver Diseases Unique to Pregnancy

Liver involvement in hyperemesis gravidum (morning sickness)

Hyperemesis gravidum is known by most people as morning sickness. It occurs during the first three months of pregnancy. In some cases, the vomiting due to morning sickness can be extremely severe, even requiring hospitalization. In such cases, liver problems are often manifested as asymptomatic elevations in blood ALT and AST activities and, sometimes, the bilirubin concentration. In severe cases the patient can become jaundiced.

Liver abnormalities associated with morning sickness are mild and of little clinical consequence. Patients who get seriously ill with this condition do so because of dehydration, not liver failure. Liver abnormalities rapidly resolve when the patient stops vomiting.

Cholestasis of pregnancy

About 1 percent of pregnant women suffer from *cholestasis of pregnancy,* which is impaired bile flow within the liver during pregnancy. The cause of this condition is not understood, but it may be related to the effects of excess estrogens on bile flow within the liver (some of the same individuals may become jaundiced while taking birth control pills). Cholestasis of pregnancy usually occurs during the last three months of pregnancy, but can sometimes occur earlier. The symptoms are pruritus (itching) in virtually all cases, and jaundice in about 25 percent. The blood bilirubin concentration and AST, ALT, alkaline phosphatase, and GGTP activities may be elevated to varying degrees.

Cholestasis of pregnancy may be unpleasant but rarely serious and never fatal. Itching may respond to treatment with cholestyramine. Several studies have reported an increased incidence of premature labor in women with cholestasis of pregnancy. A woman with this condition should therefore be monitored closely by her obstetrician.

Fatty liver of pregnancy

Fatty liver of pregnancy is one of the most serious, and often fatal, complications of pregnant women. Fortunately, it is very rare and occurs in only about 1 in 13,000 deliveries. The cause is not known but some recent studies have suggested an association with certain genetic defects in fat metabolism.

Fatty liver of pregnancy occurs during the last three months of pregnancy and is associated with sudden onset of severe liver disease. Patients may suffer from jaundice, edema, ascites, and fulminant hepatic failure. Blood tests reveal elevated aminotransferase activities. The blood bilirubin concentration is also usually elevated and prothrombin time prolonged.

Women with sudden onset severe liver disease during the third trimester must have liver biopsies to diagnose or exclude fatty liver of pregnancy. The diagnosis is made by the finding of fat (microvesicular steatosis) in hepatocytes. About 50 percent of cases are fatal to both mother and fetus. There is no treatment except for immediate delivery by cesarean section. The condition resolves after pregnancy.

Liver involvement in eclampsia and pre-eclampsia

Eclampsia and pre-eclampsia are obstetrical conditions characterized by high blood pressure and other associated abnormalities. They most frequently occur in young women during their first pregnancies. Pre-eclampsia is new onset high blood pressure during pregnancy with protein in the urine. Eclampsia is hypertension, protein in the urine, and seizures. Pre-eclampsia is a fairly common condition, and about 10 percent of women with it will have evidence of liver abnormalities in blood tests. About 5 percent will become jaundiced. Eclampsia is a rarer condition. Patients with eclampsia may develop serious liver disease. The exact causes of liver damage in pre-eclampsia and eclampsia are not known. Immediate delivery should be performed if the mother's life is in danger.

HELLP syndrome

HELLP is an abbreviation for *h*emolysis (destruction of red blood cells), *e*levated *l*iver enzymes, and *l*ow *p*latelet count. It is a relatively uncommon condition of pregnant women, usually occurring during the final three months of pregnancy. The diagnosis is made by finding the three characteristic features that define the disease (without another cause) in a pregnant woman. Mother and fetal mortality is high in HELLP syndrome. Patients should be carefully monitored and prompt delivery performed once diagnosis is made.

Pregnancy in Women with Chronic Liver Diseases

Should a woman with a chronic liver disease, who is able, become pregnant? This question falls out of the domain of science, and I cannot tell these women what to do in this regard. Some facts, however, should be considered when a woman with chronic liver disease decides to, or becomes, pregnant.

In advanced cirrhosis, pregnancy can be life threatening to the mother and fetus. Most women with very advanced cirrhosis are infertile, so pregnancy is not an issue. But elective abortion should be *considered* as an option in cases where the lives of the mother and fetus are at high risk.

Most questions about pregnancy arise in women who have either chronic hepatitis B or chronic hepatitis C without cirrhosis or early cirrhosis. In chronic hepatitis B and C, the mother must realize that there is a risk of passing on the disease to her children. This consideration aside, pregnancy is probably not very high risk in patients who do not have cirrhosis. The risk increases in women with cirrhosis, even if they do not have clinical complications.

Autoimmune hepatitis generally affects young women of childbearing potential. In autoimmune hepatitis, the drugs used to treat the disease are one issue. Prednisone and prednisolone are probably relatively safe in pregnancy, but the effects of azathioprine (Imuran) on the unborn baby are not known. If a woman with autoimmune hepatitis desires to become pregnant, azathioprine should be stopped and only prednisone or prednisolone should be used to manage the disease. If a woman with autoimmune hepatitis becomes pregnant while taking azathioprine, elective abortion should be *considered* as an option. If the woman wants to carry the pregnancy to term, all attempts should be made to stop the azathioprine as soon as possible and manage the disease with only prednisone or prednisolone for the remainder of the pregnancy. Finally, a woman with autoimmune hepatitis must realize that if a flare-up in disease activity occurs during pregnancy, her condition could become quite complicated.

Other important issues related to pregnancy are the inherited liver diseases such as Wilson disease, hemochromatosis, and alpha-1-antitrypsin deficiency. These disorders can be passed on to the baby. Professional genetic counseling should be obtained in cases where the prospective parents have questions, including situations where the disease runs in the mother's and father's families but the parents are not affected. Hemochromatosis, Wilson disease, and alpha-1-antitrypsin deficiency can theoretically be detected in the fetus prior to birth, but these tests may not be routinely available. Elective abortion is an option if a fetus is found to be affected.

CHAPTER 5

Liver Transplantation

L iver transplantation should be considered as a "life insurance policy" for individuals with chronic liver disease. Most individuals with chronic liver disease will *not* need liver transplantation. But if they do, it can save their lives. The vast majority of liver transplantation procedures are performed on patients with end-stage cirrhosis resulting from chronic liver diseases. Liver transplantation can also be performed in patients without chronic liver disease with fulminant hepatic failure.

For patients, liver transplantation can be divided into three phases: 1) pre-transplant, 2) transplant, and 3) post-transplant. The actual transplant surgery is brief compared to pre- and post-transplant periods. Patients generally have the most anxiety and questions during the pre-transplant phase. An exception, of course, is the patient with fulminant hepatic failure who may be in a coma during the pre-transplant phase.

The Pre-Transplant Evaluation

The most important aspect of liver transplantation for patients with chronic liver diseases is often for their primary doctors to know when to refer them to a transplantation center for evaluation. Good medical judgment is necessary, and the decision is not always easy. In babies, the pediatrician must readily recognize conditions such as biliary atresia that require referral to a liver specialist. In adults with chronic liver disease, deterioration is usually gradual, and the doctor must decide during many years of follow-up, when referral to a transplantation center is indicated. In cases of fulminant hepatic failure, it must be recognized immediately.

When complications of cirrhosis cannot be controlled medically, referral to a liver transplantation center is clearly indicated. The complications include worsening hepatic encephalopathy, refractory ascites, and difficulty in controlling bleeding from gastric or esophageal varices. Cachexia, or generalized wasting, sometimes becomes an unstoppable complication of cirrhosis, and transplantation should be performed before such patients literally "waste away." Other important parameters to consider include blood albumin concentration, blood bilirubin concentration, and prothrombin time. A low blood albumin concentration, rising blood bilirubin concentration, and prolonged prothrombin time indicate deterioration in liver function.

There are a few reasons *not* to refer a patient with end-stage cirrhosis for liver transplantation. Virtually no center will transplant patients who are actively abusing or dependent upon alcohol or other drugs. Such patients should first, or at least concurrently, be referred to a rehabilitation facility. Few centers will perform transplantation in patients over age seventy. At the present time, most centers will not transplant individuals with human immunodeficiency virus infection; a few have, however. Patients with metastatic cancer or other terminal diseases are also usually ineligible for liver transplantation. *If a doctor cannot determine if one of his patients is eligible for liver transplantation, he should contact a liver specialist at the nearest transplantation center to find out.*

What happens once the patient is referred to a center for liver transplantation? Usually, the patient will first be seen by a *hepatologist* or medical liver specialist. During the first visit, a transplant surgeon may also see the patient, perhaps just to introduce himself or herself. The hepatologist will take a complete medical history, review all past medical records, and perform a physical examination. The hepatologist will also order a battery of blood tests, some routine, some appropriate for the particular case, and some especially relevant to the transplant evaluation such as blood typing. The hepatologist will also answer many of the patient's and family members' questions about the liver transplantation procedure.

At the initial evaluation visit, the patient and family members will likely meet a transplant nurse coordinator. These are nurses specialized in the care of patients undergoing organ transplantation. Throughout the pre-transplantation evaluation, the patient will probably get to know the nurse coordinators best compared to any member of the transplant team. A nurse coordinator is often the first person the patient will call with questions or problems. These nurses, as their name indicates, will "coordinate" all of the multiple tests, doctor's visits, and special procedures that patients being evaluated for liver transplantation require.

At the initial consultation, the patient and/or family members may meet with a financial counselor. Liver transplantation is an expensive procedure, and the pre-transplant evaluation, surgery, and hospital stay may add up to $250,000 or more. The financial counselor will need detailed information about the patient's insurance coverage. Many major insurance policies, as well as U.S. federal-state programs such as Medicaid and Medi-Cal, will cover the costs associated with organ transplantation. Problems about financial eligibility sometimes occur with uninsured patients who do not have Medicare or Medicaid. The financial counselor may help such patients apply for benefits, or try to help arrange coverage for other expensive aspects of transplantation such as the costs of medicine after the procedure.

A patient undergoing a liver transplant evaluation will often require several radiological tests. A chest X-ray, liver ultrasound, and CAT scan will almost always be performed. The CAT scan will be done in a special way to measure the volume of the liver. This is important because a small person will need a small donor liver and a larger person a larger liver. Other radiological procedures or scans may also be performed as indicated.

As part of the transplant evaluation, the patient will also see several different doctors and health professionals. Many patients—especially older ones—will see a cardiologist for a heart evaluation. Cigarette smokers and patients with lung diseases will see a pulmonologist or medical lung specialist. Patients with kidney dysfunction will be evaluated by a nephrologist or kidney specialist. Most patients will see a psychiatrist, especially those with a history of alcohol or drug use. All patients, and usually their family members, will see a social worker for help in coping with stress and other issues associated with transplantation. Patients may also have to see a dentist to remove teeth that are decaying and could become a source of infection. Visits to other specialists or subspecialists may be scheduled as necessary.

Once the patient has undergone the necessary tests and has been evaluated by members of the transplant team and other physicians, the case is discussed by members of the transplant team in a meeting. The various doctors, nurse coordinators, financial counselors, and social workers may be asked to comment on their recommendations. Questionable test results will be discussed. After the discussion, the group as a whole makes the decision as to whether or not the patient is eligible for liver transplantation.

If the patient is deemed to be a candidate for liver transplantation, he or she is "listed" or put on the "waiting list" for a liver. Sometimes, for various medical, psychological, or social reasons, the team decides that the patient is not a transplant candidate. In rare cases, patients are not "listed" because they may not need the procedure. These patients will usually be followed by their primary doctors, sometimes in consultation with the transplant team, and reevaluated at a later date if their conditions deteriorate. Some patients are deemed ineligible for liver transplantation because other serious illnesses, such as cancer, AIDS, or heart disease, are identified during the pre-transplant evaluation. Psychological and social exclusion criteria involve active drug or alcohol use in many cases. Patients actively using drugs may be turned down for transplantation but offered another chance in the future, usually if they demonstrate at least six months of abstinence and participation in programs such as Alcoholics Anonymous.

Once a patient with liver disease is "listed" for transplantation, a waiting period begins. In the U.S., rules of the list are established by, and the list is maintained by, the United Network for Organ Sharing (UNOS). The waiting time may vary from patient to patient. Some patients who are not yet that sick may wait for a couple of years. Severely ill patients may receive livers within a few weeks. Livers are not allocated on a strict "first-come-first-serve" basis. A combination of how long the patient has been on the list and how sick he or she is determines when a donor liver will be provided. In liver transplantation, donor organs must match the recipient in blood type and size. For example, a small liver from a donor with type A blood will be transplanted into a small recipient with type A blood. To some extent, therefore, the type of liver that becomes available factors into when an individual will be transplanted. Most patients who are "listed" receive livers. Some patients, however, especially those referred late, may die before an organ becomes available.

The pre-transplant period is very different for someone with fulminant hepatic failure who does not show evidence of spontaneous recovery. In such cases, liver transplantation is the only hope for survival. Patients who have fulminant hepatic failure—who will die if not transplanted within a few days—are usually made the highest priority patients on the "waiting list."

One exception to being put on the "waiting list" would be patients who elect to have transplantation from a living-related donor. This type of transplantation is done only at some centers. In general, a parent, sibling, child, or sometimes a spouse will volunteer to donate a portion of his or her liver to the patient. Once patients are approved for living-related transplantation, the surgery can be performed when everyone is ready. In such cases, the donors may also have to undergo medical and psychosocial evaluation.

The Transplant Surgery

When a suitable donor liver becomes available, the person "whose turn it is" to receive the liver is either called at home (or "beeped" as recipients may carry pagers) or informed in his or her hospital bed that it is time for surgery. Liver transplantation is *orthotopic* in that the new liver is put in the same place as the old one. The trickiest part of the surgery is probably attaching the bile duct from the new liver to the part of the recipient's bile duct that remains in place. A major complication of liver transplant surgery is bleeding. Patients who undergo liver transplantation often have massive blood loss. Transfusion of many units of red blood cells, fresh frozen plasma, and platelets may be necessary.

After surgery, the patient is taken first to the recovery room and then the surgical intensive care unit. Most patients wake up within twenty-four hours after surgery while on a respirator. Some patients will need kidney dialysis for a few days after transplantation. The blood bilirubin concentration, ALT, and AST activities are followed carefully to establish whether or not the new liver is working. Medications to prevent *rejection* of the transplanted liver are begun at surgery and continued afterward. The concentrations of some of these medications in the blood are monitored closely and they may have to be adjusted frequently. If all goes well, a patient can leave the hospital less than two weeks after liver transplantation. Sometimes, minor (or major) complications arise that require longer hospital stays after surgery.

Post-Transplantation

Complications from surgery can occur in the immediate post-transplant period. These include bile leaks from newly sewn together bile ducts that must be treated by placement of drains by ERCP. Local wound infections and systemic infections can also occur after surgery. Bleeding is also a common occurrence after any surgical procedure. Post-operative surgical complications are usually treated successfully but they can sometimes require a return trip or two to the operating room for repair.

The major aspect of post-transplant care is to prevent organ *rejection* and infections. Rejection occurs because the recipient's immune system recognizes the grafted donor liver as foreign. A strong immune response against the organ occurs that causes it to be destroyed. Without medications to suppress the immune system, known as immunosuppressive drugs, the grafted liver would be rejected. The drugs that patients receiving organ transplants must take for the remainder of their lives are listed in Table 5.1.

Table 5.1. *Immunosuppressive drugs commonly used to prevent liver transplant rejection.*

Generic Name	Trade Name
cyclosporin A	Sandimmune®
cyclosporin A	Neoral®
tacrolimus (FK506)	Prograf®
azathioprine	Imuran®
prednisone	almost always prescribed generically
mycophenolate mofetil	CellCept®
muromonab-CD3	Orthoclone OKT®3
basiliximab	Simulect®
daclizumab	Zenapax®

Virtually all patients receiving liver transplants will take either cyclosporin A (Sandimmune or Neoral®) or tacrolimus (Prograft), which used to be called FK506. Most patients will also take prednisone and azathioprine (Imuran), which are agents that act by different mechanisms to suppress the immune system. These drugs are started immediately after transplant surgery. Each of these drugs has different side effects, and doctors may change the drugs and adjust their doses depending upon the patient's condition and adverse events experienced. These drugs are expensive, around $10,000 a year. Most importantly, *patients must take all of their immunosuppressive drugs as prescribed to prevent rejection.* Failure to take these drugs can lead to severe rejection.

After discharge from the hospital, patients will generally return to see a doctor from the transplant team at least once a week. Laboratory tests will also be checked for evidence of rejection or liver graft dysfunction. Medications may be adjusted depending upon laboratory test results. If the patient's condition remains stable, the frequency of follow-up visits will be gradually decreased.

Rejection can usually be suspected according to blood test results. Most episodes of rejection will be detected by increases in blood ALT or AST activities. Rejection can be definitively diagnosed only by liver biopsy. If blood testing suggests rejection, liver biopsy will be performed. About 75 percent of patients will experience some degree of rejection the first couple of weeks after liver transplantation. Most of these rejection episodes are mild or moderate and respond to intravenous steroids (usually methylprednisolone) followed by a brief period of increased prednisone doses. Severe rejection episodes, or those not responding to steroids, are usually treated by intravenous administration of monoclonal antibodies against lymphocytes, the white blood cells that attack the transplanted organ. In the U.S., the antibody most commonly used at present is muromonab-CD3 (Orthoclone OKT3), which recognizes a protein on the surface of lymphocytes that mediate rejection. About 10 percent of patients who undergo liver transplantation develop chronic rejection that does not respond to drugs. For these patients, a second transplant is the only available option.

Infection is another common complication after organ transplantation. Because the immune system is suppressed by drugs, post-transplant patients are at risk for infections that patients with normally functioning immune systems are not. These include infection with *Pneumocystis carinii,* which causes pneumonia, and cytomegalovirus (CMV), which causes many problems including hepatitis in the new liver. Patients usually take trimethoprim/sulfamethoxazole (Bactrim® or Septra®) to prevent Pneumocystis pneumonia. Some centers also use ganciclovir to prevent CMV infection. CMV infection can mimic rejection and the two can usually be differentiated only by liver biopsy. Many other infections that do not normally cause problems in people with normal immune systems, including those by fungi, *Mycobacterium,* and other viruses such as herpes simplex and herpes zoster, can occur.

Another concern after liver transplantation is that the original disease will recur in the new organ. Autoimmune hepatitis, primary biliary cirrhosis, and primary sclerosing cholangitis generally do not recur. If a former alcoholic does not drink, alcoholic liver disease will not occur. However, I have seen a case of alcoholic hepatitis in a patient who continued to drink after transplantation (usually such individuals will probably stop taking their immunosuppressive drugs and suffer severe rejection first). Patients who had cirrhosis from viral hepatitis B or C are at risk for the new liver to again become infected. Although the new liver is almost always reinfected with the hepatitis C virus in recipients who suffered from this disease, the degree of post-transplant hepatitis is usually mild. Severe and rapidly progressive hepatitis due to hepatitis C virus infection sometimes occurs in the transplanted liver, however. Hepatitis B virus reinfection of the new liver often leads to severe hepatitis and destruction. Fortunately, this can be prevented by drugs. Patients transplanted for cirrhosis from hepatitis B usually receive hepatitis B immune globulin (HBIG) and/or lamivudine after transplantation.

The five-year overall survival rate for patients who undergo liver transplantation at most centers is 80 to 90 percent. Many patients recover sufficiently to return to productive lives at home and work within a few months after surgery. These patients must always remember, however, to take their immunosuppressive drugs as prescribed and to follow up regularly with their doctors. They should also contact their doctors immediately should problems arise.

CHAPTER 6

Selecting a Liver Specialist

Most patients with liver diseases do not immediately seek out a liver specialist. The diagnosis of liver disease in adults is generally made first by the patient's primary doctor, usually a family practitioner or internist. In the case of children, the primary doctor is usually a family practitioner or pediatrician. Most primary doctors know how to diagnose the most common liver diseases, or at least know how to recognize a liver disease and refer the patient to a specialist for further diagnosis. Internal medicine, pediatrics, and family practice have their respective specialty boards, and in order to receive board certification in these specialties, the doctor must undergo appropriate training and pass an examination given by a specialty board. A first step in determining the qualifications of your primary doctor is to establish if she is "board certified" (having passed the specialty examination) or "board eligible" (having completed the necessary training to take the examination) in her specialty.

For further evaluation, specialized procedures, and possibly treatment, most primary doctors will refer a patient with a liver disease to a gastroenterologist. Gastroenterologists are internists or pediatricians who complete specialty training in internal medicine or pediatrics. After completing specialty training, they usually perform an additional three years of fellowship training in the subspecialty of gastroenterology. Most of this training focuses on diseases of the gastrointestinal tract, especially the esophagus, stomach, small intestine, colon, and rectum. Part of the training of all gastroenterology fellows is also focused on the diagnosis and treatment of liver diseases. There are subspecialty boards in gastroenterology, and although any doctor can call himself a "gastroenterologist," you can determine if he has actually had adequate training in this field, including some training in liver diseases, by asking if he is board certified (or board eligible) in gastroenterology. Board- certified or board-eligible pediatric or adult gastroenterologists who have trained in the U.S. have had at least some training in liver diseases.

In clinical practice, the majority of gastroenterologists devote most of their time to non-liver diseases. Some gastroenterologists take a special interest in liver diseases or *hepatology* (the study of liver diseases). Gastroenterologists who see a reasonable number of patients with liver diseases, and are skilled in diagnosis and treatment, are often referred to as hepatologists. Some of these doctors will have devoted additional time during their gastroenterology fellowship training—sometimes an entire additional year—studying liver diseases. Others who never formally trained in gastroenterology (myself included) study liver diseases sometime in their careers and become hepatologists.

Internists and pediatricians who subspecialize in hepatology only (not gastroenterology) are usually found at those academic medical centers that are closely affiliated with medical schools.

There is no official subspecialty board in hepatology. It is therefore sometimes difficult to determine if doctors who call themselves hepatologists are actually experts in liver diseases. A doctor who is a full-time faculty member at a major medical school and considered to be a liver specialist or hepatologist is probably a legitimate one. Many such doctors will have published papers in peer-reviewed journals concerning some area of liver diseases. I do not mean "articles" on the Internet, in "throwaway" medical journals, or even perhaps a book like this, but scholarly articles in medical journals that have been peer reviewed before publication. In the U.S., membership in the American Association for the Study of Liver Diseases (AASLD), a professional society, usually (but not always) indicates some degree of expertise in hepatology.

A patient with life-threatening or end-stage liver disease ultimately needs referral to a center where liver transplantation is performed (unless, of course, the patient is too sick, too old, or has a concurrent condition that excludes liver transplantation). Liver transplantation centers have medical or pediatric liver specialists with special expertise in the treatment of patients with end-stage cirrhosis or fulminant hepatic failure. Liver transplantation centers also obviously have surgeons who subspecialize in performing liver transplantation and other aspects of liver surgery. Such centers will also have doctors in a wide range of subspecialties who can handle problems that may occur in patients with end-stage liver disease, for example, kidney specialists and infectious disease specialists.

How to Find a Liver Specialist

How does a patient find a liver specialist? Usually the best source for referral is the patient's primary doctor. It is likely that the patient's primary doctor knows local specialists and subspecialists in most areas of medicine. Most primary doctors will at least know a good gastroenterologist knowledgeable in the diagnosis and treatment of liver diseases.

What if your primary doctor really does not know a liver specialist? Or what if you just do not like the specialist recommended by your primary doctor? Some organizations keep track of medical specialists. Several publications that can be found in many public libraries also list board-certified medical specialists. The American Liver Foundation is a national, voluntary, nonprofit health organization dedicated to preventing, treating, and curing liver diseases. The American Liver Foundation has several local chapters that maintain lists of liver specialists in their regions. You can reach the American Liver Foundation at:

American Liver Foundation
75 Maiden Lane, Suite 603
New York, NY 10038
1-800-GO LIVER (465-4837)
http://www.liverfoundation.org

Some patients want to see a "big expert" in liver diseases. Usually, the leading researchers and doctors in a particular field are full-time faculty members at medical schools. Before seeing such a doctor, the patient should ask if seeing one is really necessary. In most cases, the special expertise of doctors at an academic medical center is not always necessary. Also, a word of caution: "Experts" at leading medical schools often do not see patients, or will see patients only for a onetime consultation or as part of a study.

At medical centers with active liver disease research programs, there will usually be several specialists who devote most of their time to caring for patients with liver diseases. If you are fortunate enough to live near a leading medical school, and your health insurance will cover the cost, you can usually call a medical center directly for referral to a specialist. Some academic medical centers will have toll-free phone numbers for referral services. Many patients do not know this, but the best way to find a medical subspecialist is often to call the appropriate academic division directly. For example, if you are an adult with a liver disease, you can find the phone number for the office for the Division of Gastroenterology (or its equivalent, such as the Division of Digestive Diseases, Division of Liver Diseases, or Division of Hepatology) in the Department of Medicine at the nearby medical school. For a child, a similar division in the Department of Pediatrics can be contacted. You will very likely find someone there who can direct you to a specialist for your problem. Academic divisions and departments at medical schools often have websites with doctor referral information. But use caution on the Internet: *Any* doctor can advertise her practice to appear to be a world-renowned medical research institution.

Problems with HMOs

I hear many complaints from patients about how their "HMO doctors do not know enough about hepatitis C or whatever" or that their "HMO will not let me see a specialist." All that I can say is that the validity of these complaints often depends upon the HMO. Some HMOs allow access to excellent specialists who provide state-of-the-art medical care. Some, frankly, do not (there were some HMO groups in New York City whose doctors as recently as 1997 were not treating patients with chronic hepatitis C with interferon). I do not know exactly how to help a patient who perceives that his HMO doctor is not qualified to make the correct diagnosis or provide adequate treatment. One possibility is to explore legal options if your HMO or insurance provider prohibits a second opinion by a specialist. The bottom line is that life comes before money, and in some cases, a patient's only option may be to pay cash for a onetime, second opinion consultation with a liver specialist that will not be covered by her insurance. In many cases, you will be relieved to hear that your current doctor is doing everything correctly (this will probably be worth the cost of one visit). If by chance you discover your current doctor cannot handle the problem, a letter from a noted liver specialist at an academic institution explaining why you need specialized care may help in convincing your HMO to change its mind about covering the cost of outside care.

Clinical Studies

Many patients with liver diseases, especially those with chronic viral hepatitis B and C, want to be enrolled in "studies." Studies are trials of drugs or procedures on a group of patients. In good studies, some of the patients will receive a new or experimental treatment and others will receive either no treatment or the currently available one. Studies sometimes provide patients with access to new and promising drugs before they are approved by the FDA. In addition, study investigators frequently, *but not always,* have more expertise regarding the disease being studied.

Much of the recent desire for patients with liver diseases to enroll in studies has been driven by the newly available treatments for hepatitis B and C. Most of these studies are very serious clinical trials designed by academic investigators or major pharmaceutical companies. Unfortunately, some of these studies have been driven by "marketing" efforts by pharmaceutical companies to get doctors to use their products. Many of these are not studies at all but merely programs in which pharmaceutical companies pay doctors to prescribe their products to a group of patients. Some pharmaceutical sponsors will go through elaborate efforts to set up "studies" in which the companies will pay doctors to prescribe their drugs. Many "studies" of this kind are poorly designed and their results will never be published. In recent years, these kinds of "studies" have proliferated in many areas of medicine.

There are several things that patients should ask before enrolling in a study for the treatment of a liver (or any) disease. These include:

1. Where is the study taking place? Most studies that take place at medical schools or academic medical centers are probably legitimate. At these institutions they must be approved by an Institutional Review Board (IRB) that assures the trial is safe and ethical. Caution should be exercised in enrolling in studies in private doctors' offices. Some are completely legitimate, but some use so-called central IRBs that are essentially private companies that approve studies. It is not always clear if these "IRBs" impose the same standards as those at medical schools or hospitals. Ask to see proof of IRB approval before enrolling in a study.

2. Who is the study sponsor? The best studies are probably funded by the National Institutes of Health (NIH) or other government agencies, but these are few and far between. Many studies are sponsored by and/or financially supported by pharmaceutical companies and can either be "investigator initiated" or "company initiated." The distinction usually depends upon who designs the study. Some of the "company studies" may be marketing "pseudo-studies" that merely pay doctors to prescribe particular drugs. On the other hand, many "company studies" are the first and best designed trials to test a new drug. *Be more suspicious of "company studies" if a drug is already approved for the indication being studied.*

3. Who is the principal investigator of the study? A study with a full-time faculty member at a medical school as principal investigator is more likely (but not always) a better choice than a study conducted in the office of a doctor who does not have a medical school affiliation.

4. Ask your doctor! Never enroll in a clinical trial without discussing it first with your doctor.

Most studies will *not* involve new drugs conducted by professors at the best medical schools and funded by the NIH. On the other hand, most studies will not be poorly designed marketing efforts to induce doctors to prescribe particular drugs. They are usually something in between. Just remember to make certain beforehand that the study is IRB approved. Do some homework and find out the reputations of the sponsor and principal investigator. And check with your doctor before enrolling.

CHAPTER 7

Living with Liver Disease

P eople with liver disease must live with their illness. This is
sometimes difficult for their doctors to realize. It is often
difficult for family members and friends to realize. It is also
sometimes difficult for patients to accept.

It is difficult to give any specific recommendations about living with liver disease. First of all, there are many different
chronic liver diseases, and the outlook for each is different. The
prognosis for different patients with the same disease can also
vary tremendously. Most patients with chronic hepatitis B or
chronic hepatitis C will live full and essentially normal lives
while others will develop cirrhosis and possibly liver cancer.
*Perhaps scariest of all is that you often cannot be sure what will
happen to you.*

In an attempt to provide some general rules about living
with liver disease, it is important to realize that some patients
have very special needs. Most important to consider are patients
with liver diseases who are *actively* abusing alcohol or other

drugs or are dependent upon alcohol or other substances. The social and psychological issues of patients who are substance abusers make their priorities quite different. Another small group of patients having special considerations are those with advanced cancer involving the liver. Such patients should probably seek out cancer support groups and foundations such as the American Cancer Society for information. Finally, young children have special needs that are different from adults. There are several support groups devoted to children with liver disease, and pediatricians should also prove helpful in these instances.

I discuss some general guidelines that I think will help all people in "living with liver disease." I then discuss the special needs of patients actively using alcohol or drugs. At the end of this section, I provide a list (admittedly incomplete) of patient organizations that provide access to support groups and information.

General Guidelines

Many patients live with their liver disease appropriately and need very little outside support. Others are terrified. What I find terrifies most patients is:

- Uncertainty. Most patients do not know if they will develop serious complications from their disease or if it will shorten their lives.
- Fear. Many patients fear that liver disease will kill them.
- Lack of information. Many patients are not well informed about their disease and do not understand it.

- Misinformation and misunderstanding. Many patients hear things about liver diseases (often on the Internet) that are not true or relevant to their cases.

Uncertainty

Most patients with chronic liver disease live full and normal lives. Some, such as those with primary biliary cirrhosis, will invariably progress. Those with chronic viral hepatitis may or may not have their condition progress to cirrhosis. Rarely can a patient with chronic liver disease be told with 99 percent certainty whether the disease will progress to end-stage cirrhosis or not. Patients with chronic liver disease should not fixate on the worst outcomes; those occur in a minority of cases only. *Patients with chronic liver diseases should live and plan for full and exciting lives!* They should follow up regularly with a knowledgeable doctor and discuss all their problems and concerns. And just in case things do worsen, a patient with a chronic liver disease should realize that transplantation is a "life insurance policy" and keep this in the back of her mind.

Fear

Most patients with chronic liver disease will *not* die from it. However, the uncertainty discussed above will often breed fear. Sometimes this is difficult to overcome and patients should discuss these issues with their doctor. If fear is excessive, they should consider consultation with a health professional (psychiatrist, psychologist, social worker) who can help. Finally, there are many legitimate support groups for patients with liver disease, some of which are listed at the end of this chapter.

Lack of Information and Misinformation

Ask your doctor! Ask your doctor! Ask your doctor! If you do not trust your doctor, obtain a second opinion from another doctor. Despite all of the patient information currently available, including my book and a plethora of Websites, only a doctor who knows the patient well can answer specific questions regarding diagnosis, treatment, and prognosis in a specific case. Use books such as this one, reliable Internet resources, and information from patient organizations to *help* you understand your disease. *Never* use these resources as a substitute for good medical care.

Be careful of misinformation, especially on the Internet. On the World Wide Web, anyone can appear to be an expert. Be leery of Websites, books, "doctors," and other sources claiming "new" or "miracle" cures for liver diseases.

Don't believe what you hear about "alternative," "herbal," or "holistic" remedies. Believe me, if such remedies or methods had been subjected to rigorous scientific testing, mainstream physicians and scientists would take note. None of these remedies has yet been subjected to scientific scrutiny or tested in controlled clinical trials. Milk thistle and its "active ingredient" silymarin have been promoted by fans of alternative medicine—and even some mainstream doctors—as compounds for general "liver health." They have also been promoted as cures for virtually every known liver disease. Despite the hype, to the best of my knowledge, *milk thistle or silymarin has never been shown to be effective in a controlled clinical trial for any liver disease.* Furthermore, these and many other "herbal" or "alternative" remedies have not even been proven safe for patients with liver disorders. So be careful about what you hear without doing further research on your own!

Trust what you hear from your doctor or legitimate patient organizations such as the American Liver Foundation. Take any other information with a grain of salt. If you want to research something, go to the library and search the medical literature or conduct a search on the Internet (try Pub Med at http://www. ncbi.nlm.nih.gov/PubMed/). Bring articles to your doctor and seek help from an expert when trying to understand complex medical issues.

Patients Actively Abusing Alcohol or Other Substances

Alcohol is the number one cause of liver disease in the Western world. In the same countries, intravenous drug use is also a major risk factor for hepatitis B and hepatitis C. For these reasons, a large number of patients with liver disease have substance abuse or substance dependence disorders. *For patients with active substance use disorders, the number one priority is to deal with the substance disorder.* I cannot emphasize this enough. It applies to the patient with alcoholic hepatitis who is finally discharged from the hospital, the alcoholic with cirrhosis who cannot be considered for liver transplantation while drinking, or the heroin addict with chronic hepatitis C who wants treatment. Even for those with cirrhosis and end-stage liver disease, treating their drug use is the number one priority. Individuals who need liver transplantation to survive will almost *never* receive a transplant if they are actively abusing drugs or alcohol.

All of the information for patients not actively abusing alcohol or drugs also applies to the person with liver disease who is actively using these substances. However, *dealing with the substance disorder is always the number one priority* and must be emphasized separately from everything else. Some general guidelines for alcohol or substance users with liver diseases follow:

Rehabilitation

Many individuals with drug or alcohol abuse or dependency disorders require inpatient rehabilitation—usually a one-month voluntary stay in a facility where intensive treatment is directed at the substance disorder.

Alcoholics Anonymous and Narcotics Anonymous

Alcoholics Anonymous (AA) is an informal society of more than 2 million recovered alcoholics in the U.S., Canada, and other countries. These men and women meet in local groups ranging in size from a handful in some localities to many hundreds in larger communities. Narcotics Anonymous (NA) is a similar society for individuals with other drug abuse or dependency disorders. Individuals with liver diseases and alcohol or other substance abuse disorders should participate in AA or NA, respectively. *Anyone can contact AA or NA. You do not need a referral.* (See Appendix B for additional resources.)

Alcoholics Anonymous World Services, Inc.
P.O. Box 459
New York, NY 10163
(212) 870-3400
http://www.alcoholics-anonymous.org

Outside of the U.S. or Canada, write or call the AA General Service Office closest to you.

Narcotics Anonymous World Services
P.O. Box 9999
Van Nuys, CA 91409
(818) 773-9999
fax (818) 700-0700

In Europe:

48 Rue de l'êté/Zomerstraat
B-1050 Brussels, Belgium
32-2-646-6012
fax 32-2-649-9239
http://www.na.org

Concurrent Medical Care

The sick person with a drug or alcohol abuse or dependence disorder will also require medical care for other conditions while in a rehabilitation program or attending AA or NA meetings. The patient should follow up with a doctor regularly who understands their treatment needs. Many rehabilitation programs also offer medical services. Some patients with substance abuse disorders may also benefit from psychiatric care, and patients should discuss referral to a psychiatrist, perhaps one specializing in substance abuse disorders, with their primary care physician or liver specialist.

Family Support

Family members and friends should be supportive of an individual's commitment to treat a substance abuse disorder. Sometimes it can be incredibly stressful, especially if a loved one refuses treatment and continues to abuse alcohol or drugs. If family members or friends are having a difficult time with a loved one who abuses alcohol, they can contact Al-Anon, a worldwide organization that offers a self-help recovery program for families and friends of alcoholics whether or not the alcoholic seeks help or even recognizes the existence of a drinking problem. Al-Anon also has a division called Alateen for younger members. In the U.S. or Canada, you can call 1-800-344-2666 for the location of an Al-Anon or Alateen meeting near you.

Al-Anon also maintains a Website at http://www.Al-Anon-Alateen.org where you can find information in numerous languages and contact information for many countries.

The patient with liver disease and a substance abuse or dependence disorder has two problems to deal with. The special needs of these patients require medical care, frequently psychiatric treatment, *self-help,* and participation in programs such as Alcoholics Anonymous or Narcotics Anonymous. In addition, the advice for patients not abusing alcohol or other substances is relevant to these individuals. Most important, individuals with substance abuse disorders, as well as their doctors, family members, and friends, must realize that treatment of these disorders is every bit as serious an issue—and sometimes more serious—as treatment of the liver disease.

Children

Depending upon their age and sophistication, children will have different degrees of insight into their medical conditions. What is most important for parents to understand is that children with chronic liver disease should, in most cases, be treated like all other kids! Most can go to school, play, and participate in sports. Most will lead long and normal lives and probably not suffer from complications of liver disease.

I receive many inquiries from parents whose children have liver problems. A very common concern comes from parents whose child is chronically infected with the hepatitis B virus. These parents often think that it is the end of the world for their child. However, the parents should realize that most children with liver disease will do well. Most importantly, as for adults, they should plan for their children to lead full and normal lives and remember that liver transplantation is an "insurance policy" if needed. For children who are very ill or who need transplantation, several support groups are available.

Support Groups

I have listed just a few support groups for patients with liver diseases that I feel are reputable. I apologize in advance to all of the legitimate support groups that I have excluded. The ones listed here probably have the greatest national presence in the U.S. Smaller regional groups are excluded from this list. (See Appendix B for additional resources.)

For All Patients with Liver Diseases:
American Liver Foundation
75 Maiden Lane, Suite 603
New York, NY 10038
1-800-GO LIVER (465-4837)
http://www.liverfoundation.org

For Patients with Alcohol or Drug Problems:
Alcoholics Anonymous (AA) World Services, Inc.
P.O. Box 459
New York, NY 10163
(212) 870-3400
http://www. alcoholics-anonymous.org

Narcotics Anonymous World Services
P.O. Box 9999
Van Nuys, CA 91409
(818) 773-9999
http://www.na.org

Liver Transplantation and Childhood Liver Diseases:
American Share Foundation
15314 Gault Street, #314
Van Nuys, CA 91406
(818) 994-6848
http://www.asf.org/

Organ Transplant Fund, Inc.
1102 Brookfield, Suite 202
Memphis, TN 38119
1-800-489-3863
http://www.otf.org

Viral Hepatitis:
Hepatitis B Coalition Immunization Action Coalition
1573 Selby Avenue, Suite 229
St. Paul, MN 55104-6328
(612) 647-9009
http://www.immunize.org

Hepatitis Foundation International
30 Sunrise Terrace
Cedar Grove, NJ 07009-1423
(201) 239-1035 or 1-800-891-0707
http://www.hepfi.org

CHAPTER 8

Research and the Future

Perhaps the most exciting aspect of modern medicine is that basic scientific advances made in the laboratory will lead to new diagnostic methods and treatments of diseases. Since the revolution in molecular biology and the emergent discipline of biotechnology that was built upon it, the amount of time it takes for discoveries in the laboratory to be translated to a patient's bedside has decreased dramatically. One of the best examples of how the emerging discipline of biotechnology has had a tremendous impact on a human disease, in fact, concerns liver disease. This disease is hepatitis C.

The hepatitis C virus was first discovered in 1989. Before that time, it could not be diagnosed and the blood supply could not be adequately screened. Now, diagnosis and treatment of chronic hepatitis C has literally become an entire "industry." Several companies produce various diagnostic assays. In the U.S., three pharmaceutical companies currently have medications approved for the treatment of chronic hepatitis C and many more have drugs in the "pipeline." Researchers in academic laboratories and companies are trying to better understand how this virus infects and damages liver cells and are working to develop new methods to stop infection and replication.

Surveying all the different liver diseases, it is unlikely that our fight against all of them will progress at equal rates. I am optimistic that, in the very near future, highly effective treatments will exist for many liver diseases. Tops on my list for major advances in the next decade are the developments of specific medications to treat chronic viral hepatitis. I also think that better treatments may evolve for genetic diseases such as hemochromatosis and Wilson disease now that the genes for these disorders have been identified and they can be understood at the molecular level. It is also probable that transplant immunology will advance, making liver transplantation safer and more effective.

While still optimistic, I am concerned that the understanding of some liver diseases will lag and effective treatments will not be developed. The "autoimmune" liver disease will probably remain a major challenge without a significant breakthrough in treatment during the next few years. I do not think that significant advances will be made in slowing the liver's response to chronic injury, namely the scarring and abnormal regeneration of the liver that leads to development of cirrhosis. In some instances, socioeconomic factors will slow progress in our fight against liver diseases. An example is hepatitis B. At the present time, there are effective vaccines that could theoretically eradicate this virus. If cheap vaccines are not distributed to the underdeveloped countries of the world where hepatitis B virus infection is endemic, however, eradicating this disease will remain a dream.

I would like to provide some of my views on research and the *near* future for patients with liver diseases. I do not have a crystal ball, and basic scientific discoveries that are made today may change my opinions tomorrow. Based upon what I know today, however, I will speculate on where I think some of the most promising breakthroughs will occur during the next decade.

Treatment for Viral Hepatitis

Until recently, there were no specific drugs to treat viral infections. When a virus infects a host cell, it must use some of the host cell's own machinery to replicate. For this reason, drugs that attack viruses and do not simultaneously harm the host cells have been very difficult to design.

One of the first breakthroughs in designing specific antiviral drugs came against the human immunodeficiency virus (HIV). HIV causes AIDS. At the time the virus was discovered in 1980, progression of HIV infection to AIDS was almost a certainty with a life expectancy of about eighteen months once it was diagnosed. In the fifteen years or so since HIV was discovered, however, major strides have been made to allow people infected with this virus to live long and productive lives.

The development of HIV protease inhibitors and DNA polymerase inhibitors has led to so-called *combination therapy*. This has revolutionized the treatment of HIV-infected individuals. Combination therapy utilizes drugs having different mechanisms of action at the same time. If the virus develops resistance to one drug by mutation, the other drugs will theoretically remain effective. Furthermore, a combination of drugs working at two distinct targets may be more effective in inhibiting viral replication than any one drug against any one target. Combination therapy is not a new idea in medicine and it has been used for some time in cancer chemotherapy and treatment of bacterial infections such as tuberculosis. However, the explosion in research on HIV made this the first *virus* against which combination therapy has been successfully utilized. By taking two DNA polymerase inhibitors and a protease inhibitor, many patients with HIV infection are now living longer and not developing AIDS.

I predict that in the next several years combination therapy with more *specific* drugs will be available for the treatment of hepatitis B and hepatitis C. Interferon alpha and ribavirin are effective drugs for viral hepatitis and result in "cures" in some people, but they are *not* specific. Interferon alpha is a natural product made by your body that stimulates the immune system to fight viral infections. The theory behind giving excessive amounts of interferon is that it helps your own body attack the hepatitis B and hepatitis C virus. Unfortunately, interferon alpha has other effects. They are readily apparent from the unpleasant symptoms that many individuals suffer while taking it. Ribavirin is a nonspecific drug that "looks like" a molecular building block essential to viral metabolism. Combined with interferon, it helps fight the hepatitis C virus but it does not *specifically* attack any viral proteins.

More specific drugs are already being utilized in clinical trials for hepatitis B. Lamivudine is a DNA polymerase inhibitor approved for treatment of hepatitis B that also inhibits the HIV DNA polymerase. Several other compounds that similarly inhibit the hepatitis B virus DNA polymerase are also under investigation in clinical trials.

One problem with having only one available inhibitor of the hepatitis B viral DNA polymerase is that the virus can develop resistance by mutation. HIV and hepatitis B virus both develop resistance to lamivudine by similar mechanisms. In HIV infection, two protease inhibitors, lamivudine and AZT, for example, are used together, hence making resistance to both a less likely occurrence. When additional inhibitors against the hepatitis B virus become available, combination therapy with two or more will probably become the standard of care to treat infection. I think that in the next several years, treatment of hepatitis B virus infection will be conducted using combination therapy with one or two or more DNA polymerase inhibitors and possibly even interferon alpha.

What about hepatitis C? My prediction is that specific drugs for the treatment of hepatitis C will be developed and tested in clinical trials within the decade. In the past few years, the crystal structures of the hepatitis C virus NS3 protease, NS4A protease cofactor, and N3S RNA-helicase have been determined. These proteins carry out specific functions necessary for virus replication. If the functions of these viral proteins are inhibited, the virus cannot replicate. Crystal structures of proteins provide chemists with "pictures" of the molecules. By looking at these pictures, chemists can design drugs that may bind to and inhibit them. This method is called "rational drug design" because, rather than trying millions of compounds in potluck fashion, drugs can be synthesized based upon knowledge of the target's structure. Rational drug design can be combined with another type of methodology called "combinatorial chemistry" in which a "library" of thousands of structurally similar molecules is synthesized and tested against the target. "High throughput screening" can be performed in part by robots to speed the screening process. By combining rational drug design and combinatorial chemistry, inhibitors of these viral proteins can be rapidly identified. Many pharmaceutical and biotechnology companies are currently doing exactly this to develop drugs against hepatitis C virus.

The future treatment of chronic hepatitis C virus infection will probably be combination therapy with helicase, protease,

RNA polymerase inhibitors, and possibly other novel drugs. Interferon, possibly at lower doses, may be used along with these more specific compounds. Because hepatitis C is a slowly progressive chronic disease, people with this disorder who do not respond to currently available treatments should be optimistic that other treatments will be available during their lifetime.

Vaccination for Chronic Viral Hepatitis

Effective vaccines for hepatitis A and hepatitis B already exist. Universal vaccination with hepatitis B virus has already been shown to decrease the incidence of liver cancer in Taiwan. This sounds revolutionary, but it is true: A vaccine that prevents cancer. It is a shame that hepatitis B vaccination is least available in the parts of the world where it is needed most. Universal vaccination, such as that for smallpox, could eradicate hepatitis B completely. Unfortunately, socioeconomic and not scientific factors will make this unlikely in the near future. The same holds true for hepatitis A.

A vaccine against hepatitis C virus may be difficult to develop as there are several different genotypes and the virus can mutate into quasispecies that are not recognized by the immune system. However, novel scientific research may lead to a vaccine by the end of the next decade. Unfortunately, if realized, a hepatitis C vaccine may remain a commodity for citizens of wealthy nations only—and not be available in other parts of the world where it is needed.

Inherited Diseases

"Human Genome Project" and "genomics" are virtually household terms. Sometime early in the twenty-first century, the entire human genome will be sequenced. This means that every gene that encodes every human protein will be identified and the basic structures of encoded proteins known. Concerning liver diseases, the impact of this type of work has already been realized. In the 1990s, the genes responsible for Wilson disease and hereditary hemochromatosis were identified. Screening tests for these diseases are now possible. Furthermore, the basic structures of encoded proteins are known and their functions are being studied in the laboratory. Such studies should lead to drugs or other methods of treatment, such as gene therapy, for these genetic disorders. For example, recent studies have shown how the hemochromatosis protein regulates uptake of iron by cells. Knowledge of these mechanisms can lead to the development of drugs having the same functions in patients with the disease who lack functional protein.

Although I think that the "autoimmune" liver diseases will not benefit from major breakthroughs during their treatment in the next decade, the rapidly growing field of genomics may have some impact on these diseases, too. They are not "inherited" in the traditional sense, however; individuals probably inherit many different genes that "predispose" them to acquiring these diseases. When the mapping of all human genes is completed early in the next millennium, it may be possible to identify which genes predispose people to these autoimmune diseases. The identification of these genes may lead to breakthroughs in understanding what goes wrong with the immune system in individuals who have them.

Transplant Immunology

Liver transplantation is a lifesaving procedure for those with end-stage cirrhosis or fulminant hepatic failure. The major problem most patients face after liver or other organ transplantation is that their own immune systems recognize the transplanted tissues as foreign and reject them. At the present time, this problem is solved using drugs that suppress parts of the immune system. These drugs not only prevent transplant rejection but also suppress the immune system so that it is less able to fight off certain types of infections that are of little or no consequence to an otherwise healthy person. Long-term suppression of the immune system by these drugs also makes that patient susceptible to certain types of cancer as the "anticancer surveillance" of the immune system is partially disabled.

Over the past several years, an explosion of knowledge has taken place concerning our fundamental understanding of the immune system. Over the next several years, specific drugs that prevent the immune system from attacking the transplanted organ may be developed. For example, drugs that block the "foreign" molecules on the transplanted organ from being recognized by the host's immune system will prevent organ rejection but not inhibit its ability to fight infection or cancer. I think that these drugs may not be available tomorrow but perhaps near the end of the next decade.

Another hot topic in organ transplantation is *xenotransplantation*—where organs are transplanted between species. If xenotransplantation is ever widely employed (ethical and scientific issues remain), it is likely to have a major impact on liver transplantation because donor organs are at a shortage in many parts of the world. Xenotransplantation is most often discussed concerning the organs of pigs and humans. In general, a pig liver would be instantly rejected when transplanted into a human because the immune system detects certain proteins on the surface of pig cells to be foreign. Current immunosuppressive drugs cannot stop this intense reaction against such foreign proteins. However, advances in genetic engineering and cloning large animals (like Dolly the sheep) will theoretically make it possible to block the expression of foreign proteins on cells, and consequently clone large numbers of pigs that lack these proteins. Thus, entire farms could be established where cloned pigs are raised to provide organs for human transplantation. This may sound like something out of a futuristic science fiction novel; however, scientifically it will likely be possible in the next few years.

In addition to the ethical issues of breeding pigs to produce organs (many of you have probably eaten pork chops), there are concerns that pig pathogens may gain access to the human population by transplantation and mutate to new forms that will then become human pathogens. For example, if a pig virus is transplanted to a human host, and the host is receiving immunosuppressive drugs to prevent rejection of the transplanted liver, that pig virus may replicate in the host and mutate to a form that can infect human cells. The fear is that this may allow for the "evolution" of novel viruses that can cause disease in humans and become widespread in the population. At present, many scientists feel that there should be a moratorium on xenotransplantation until these possibilities are excluded. Others feel that the risk is small. Some biotechnology companies are already gearing up to produce animal organs for transplantation into humans.

Supporting Research

Compared to funding for AIDS, cancer, and heart disease, funding for liver diseases is very low in the U.S. Despite tremendous fundraising efforts, the American Liver Foundation can fund only about $1 million worth of research projects per year. By contrast, the average one-year budget of a *single grant* funded by the American Cancer Society is over $100,000. Cancer and heart disease kill more Americans than liver disease, but liver disease research remains abysmally funded by any measure.

Many people with liver disease or their family members are interested in supporting relevant research. There are a few things that everyone should realize when considering how to support liver disease research:

1. Most medical research in the U.S. is supported by the National Institutes of Health (NIH). Much NIH-funded research, despite being called "cancer research," "heart research," or whatever, is basic and will have implications for all human diseases. If you want to support broad, basic medical research, call, write, or send e-mail to your congressional representatives to broadly increase funding for the NIH.
2. If you donate money to a legitimate foundation such as the American Liver Foundation (ALF), do not worry about it being "targeted" to a specific disease or scientist. This decision is better left to scientists on ALF advisory boards who make these decisions and know which areas of research, and investigators, are likely to benefit from increased funding.
3. More money is needed for basic laboratory research. Pharmaceutical companies spend billions of dollars every year

developing drugs. They also spend billions supporting clinical trials. Relatively speaking, basic research—that with the most promise for the future—is poorly funded. You will get much more bang for your buck by supporting basic, fundamental research.

If you, a family member, or friend suffers from a liver disease, you will benefit from basic research that is taking place now. Stay optimistic about your future.

Frequently Asked Questions

As a liver specialist and researcher who maintains a popular World Wide Website on liver diseases, I receive thousands of e-mail questions from patients. Over the years, I have noticed many similar or identical questions. Hopefully, the answers to most of them will be obvious to anyone who reads this book. Nevertheless, to emphasize and clarify issues of common concern, I have decided to include a list of fifteen questions that people ask me most often about liver diseases.

Q: I was just denied insurance because my "liver enzymes" are elevated. What does this mean?

A: There are several laboratory blood tests that are commonly referred to as "liver enzymes." These include the alanine aminotransferase (ALT), aspartate aminotransferase (AST), alkaline phosphatase, and gamma-glutamyltranspeptidase (GGTP) activities. There are *many* causes of elevations of these enzyme activities in the blood and *only a doctor who knows the complete history* *and examines the patient can make a diagnosis.* In general, elevations in blood ALT and AST activities indicate inflammation of the liver (hepatitis) or destruction of liver cells from other causes. The most common liver disorders that cause ALT and AST activities to be elevated are probably alcohol-related liver disease, chronic hepatitis C, chronic hepatitis B, prescription drugs, and fatty liver. There are other possible causes, however. In general, elevations in alkaline phosphatase and GGTP activities indicate bile duct diseases; however, they may be elevated in other liver diseases, too. Serum GGTP activity alone may become elevated from heavy alcohol drinking, consumption of other drugs, or for no apparent reason in some normal individuals. Blood alkaline phosphatase activity may be elevated in bone disorders in the absence of liver disease. Elevations in any of these enzymes are not diseases *per se,* but indicate that something may be wrong. Anyone learning about "abnormal liver function tests" or "liver enzymes" should *see a doctor for a diagnosis.*

Q: What do you think of milk thistle (silymarin) for my liver disease?

A: In the world of so-called alternative or herbal medicine, silymarin, which is present in milk thistle, has become the substance to help anyone with any liver disease. Some individuals even advocate taking this to "keep the liver healthy." In short, there is *no* scientific evidence that silymarin or milk thistle is an effective treatment or preventative agent for any liver disease.

First, there should be a sound scientific basis for the effectiveness of any substance to treat a disease or condition. This usually results from laboratory studies or studies on animals. To the best of my knowledge, there is no reproducible laboratory research proving that silymarin does anything to protect the liver or improve any model disease. Next, before any compound can be considered effective in humans it must also be tested in clinical trials. The gold-standard clinical trial is randomized, double-blind, placebo-controlled. In such a trial, many subjects are randomly assigned to receive either an investigational new drug, a placebo (dummy drug), or an older established therapy if one exists. Neither the attending doctors nor the patients know which they are receiving (this is what "double-blind" means). All patients are monitored for adverse events and responses to treatment. Responses must be defined before the study begins to prevent looking backward for apparently effective results. At the end of the study, it is disclosed which individuals received the new drug and which did not. Adverse events and responses to treatment are compared between the two groups and a statistical analysis is then performed to establish with the highest degree of probability that any detected differences are real and not a result of chance. Results from studies such as these are what the FDA usually wants to see before it approves a drug for public consumption. To the best of my knowledge, there are no randomized, double-blind, placebo-controlled studies of silymarin for any liver disease. Therefore, the effectiveness of this compound or, for that matter, its potential dangers, has not yet been established.

Q: My relative or friend drinks excessively. He has symptoms of liver disease but refuses to get help. What can I do?

A: This is an unfortunate and common situation. A relative or friend can suggest, even insist, that a patient seek medical help for any disease—including substance dependence—but cannot force the individual to seek help. The best approach is to probably suggest that the sick individual see a doctor to help him feel better. Regarding alcohol abuse, the friend or family member can also suggest that the individual go to an Alcoholics

Anonymous meeting. Unfortunately, these approaches often do not work, especially with substance dependence.

Al-Anon (and Alateen for younger individuals) is a world-wide organization offering self-help programs for families and friends of alcoholics whether or not the alcoholic seeks help or even recognizes the existence of a drinking problem. If a friend or family member of an individual with alcohol abuse or alcohol dependence needs help and support, he or she should contact Al-Anon or Alateen (http://www.Al-Anon-Alateen.org/).

Q: My doctor told me I have hepatitis C. Do I need a liver biopsy?

A: Individuals who are newly diagnosed with chronic hepatitis C almost always ask if they need a liver biopsy. There is no absolute right or wrong answer to this question, but I'll try to explain the reason why *most* liver specialists will recommend a liver biopsy for *most* patients with chronic hepatitis C. Let's first deal with the issue of patients in whom liver biopsy may not change things that much. For example, percutaneous liver biopsy is high risk in someone with cirrhosis, a low platelet count, and elevated prothrombin time. If the presence of cirrhosis is already obvious, liver biopsy should be performed in these patients only if the information obtained will somehow influence the outcome. Liver biopsy would probably have to be performed by an alternative approach such as a laparoscope. If this patient has strong evidence of hepatitis C (history of a risk factor and positive laboratory tests), biopsy is not necessary to confirm the diagnosis. Because it is already obvious that the patient has cirrhosis, biopsy is not necessary to establish the presence of fibrosis or cirrhosis or how the degree of inflammation will influence prognosis. Biopsy may be necessary only if a different diagnosis is possible or if a tumor is suspected.

Liver biopsy may also not be necessary in individuals where liver disease is not a primary problem For example, there is probably no need to assess the prognosis of a patient with hepatitis C if she has another concurrent disease. The prognostic information obtained by liver biopsy may also not prove useful in an elderly individual. After all, why perform a liver biopsy in an eighty-year-old with hepatitis C?

But what about most patients with a clinical and laboratory diagnosis of hepatitis C and no other medical contraindications to the procedure? In almost all such cases, liver biopsy provides essential data that cannot be obtained by any other test. *Most* liver specialists would advocate liver biopsy in such individuals. First of all, in relatively healthy individuals without complications of cirrhosis, known bleeding disorders, or other medical problems, the risk of complications from liver biopsy is very small. In exchange for this very small risk, the biopsy will provide critical information, especially regarding prognosis and possible response to treatment. Only liver biopsy can establish for certain if most patients with chronic hepatitis C have cirrhosis. The degree of inflammation and fibrosis on biopsy also provide important prognostic information. No fibrosis and minimal inflammation correlate to a good prognosis. The absence of cirrhosis, significant scarring, and minimal inflammation also correlate to better response to treatment. Hence, the information obtained by liver biopsy is extremely useful in most individuals with chronic hepatitis C.

Q: How does someone get on the list for a liver transplantation and how long is the list?

A: Patients, and even their primary doctors, do *not* decide who is eligible for liver transplantation (at least in the U.S.). This decision can be made only at medical centers where transplantation is performed. It depends upon a comprehensive evaluation by hepatologists, surgeons, psychiatrists, social workers, and sometimes other medical subspecialists. The decision is then made by consensus after the findings of each specialist are considered. Thus, the only way a patient can become a candidate for liver transplantation is to be evaluated at a center where liver transplantation is performed.

Once the patient is approved, he is put on a "waiting list" for transplantation. The "list" is composed of the names of all individuals who have been deemed eligible for transplantation at a particular center. Several factors are taken into account concerning a given patient's priority to receive an available donor liver. These factors include the amount of waiting time (depending upon how many individuals are currently on the list) and the urgency for transplantation (how long a patient can survive without a new liver). In general, waiting time is determined by a combination of how sick the patient is and how long the patient has been waiting.

Q: What can I do to keep my liver healthy?

A: Many people seem to believe that there is some sort of "healthy liver diet" or "healthy liver lifestyle." These beliefs probably derive from so-called alternative or holistic medical practices. Many alternative or holistic products include preparations for a healthy liver, heart, kidney, and so forth. Milk thistle or silymarin (see second question) is sometimes considered to be a product that "strengthens" the liver or keeps it healthy.

In truth, there are no substances or diets for a "healthy liver." In general, a lifestyle conducive to general good health is good for the liver. All individuals should minimize fat in their diets and try to maintain an ideal weight by watching what foods they eat and exercising regularly. This will avoid accumulation of fat in the liver just as it will in all other parts of the body. Alcohol consumption *in moderation* will *not* damage a healthy liver and common sense should be used. Finally, risk factors for conditions that can damage the liver should be avoided. These include excessive alcohol consumption, intravenous drug use, and the use of drugs, herbs, or "remedies" that may be toxic.

Q: I have pain in the right side of my abdomen. Could it be my liver?

A: My answer to this question is that pain in the abdomen may be attributed to many sources and only a doctor who examines the patient can determine the cause. Usually, individuals with chronic liver diseases do not have pain in the area of the liver. However, acute liver inflammation, tumors, and other mass lesions can cause pain if they irritate the liver capsule. Pain in the right upper portion of the abdomen is caused more often by disorders of the gallbladder, colon, or even the diaphragm than by diseases of the liver.

Q: My ultrasound/CT scan/biopsy/etc., shows [whatever]. What does it mean?

A: Many patients with liver diseases are deeply concerned about one particular test result. It is usually what they consider the "big" test or any test that is not routine. Frequently, people are concerned about a pathologist's report of a liver biopsy or a radiologist's report about a CAT scan or ultrasound scan. All I can say is that in most cases, the results of one individual test are meaningless without knowing the patient's complete medical history. Concerns about a specific test must be directed to a doctor who has examined the patient and knows the entire case history.

Q: I've just been diagnosed with a chronic liver disease; is it all over or will I get cirrhosis?

A: Most individuals with chronic liver diseases live full and normal lives. Most individuals with alcoholic liver disease who do not yet have advanced cirrhosis will get better if they stop drinking. Even without treatment, *most* individuals with chronic hepatitis B and chronic hepatitis C do not develop cirrhosis in their lifetime. Some chronic liver diseases, such as primary biliary cirrhosis, invariably lead to cirrhosis; progression may be slow, however, and patients may have a normal life span and die of other natural causes before developing complications from liver disease. Unfortunately, it is often difficult to predict which individual patients with chronic liver diseases will progress to cirrhosis and which ones will not. Perhaps most importantly, measures can be taken to prevent the chance of progression to chronic liver disease in *most* patients. Individuals with alcoholic liver disease must stop drinking. Chronic hepatitis B or hepatitis C can be treated with alpha interferons and other drugs. Auto-immune hepatitis responds to treatment with steroids and azathioprine. Ursodiol may slow the progression of primary biliary cirrhosis. Effective treatments are also available for hemochromatosis and Wilson disease. Finally, liver transplantation can be looked upon as a kind of "insurance policy" and lifesaving treatment of last resort for patients with chronic liver diseases that progress to end-stage cirrhosis. All things considered, most patients with chronic liver diseases should *not* die from them.

Q: What are lesions (spots) on the liver?

A: For some reason, lots of people ask me about "lesions (or spots) on the liver." My guess is that these questions stem from abnormal ultrasound or CAT scans that detect a mass, cyst, or other abnormality in the liver. Radiologists and other doctors often call these "lesions" and frequently tell patients that "lesions" were found in the liver on the test that was performed. These "lesions" can be *many* different things, some benign and some very serious. So "lesions on the liver" is *not* a diagnosis but merely a statement indicating that something was detected in the liver—usually on a radiological test—that normally should not be there. Further tests, frequently biopsy, may be required to determine what the "lesions" are.

Q: A friend has cancer of the liver. What can she do now?

A: *Liver cancer* is not a very specific term. First, the type of liver cancer must be specified. *Hepatocellular carcinoma* is primary liver cancer or a cancer that arises in the liver. The cell of origin appears to be the hepatocyte. Hepatocellular carcinoma is rather rare in the U.S., but it is a leading cause of cancer death worldwide. It almost always occurs in the U.S. in individuals with cirrhosis. Around the world, chronic infection with hepatitis B virus is the major risk factor. Cancers can also arise in the liver from the bile duct cells and are called *cholangiocarcinomas*.

Most "liver cancers" in the U.S. and other Western countries are *metastatic* carcinomas. Carcinomas arise in solid organs from cells of the epithelial type. Carcinomas arise in almost any other organ, common examples being the colon, rectum, pancreas, lung, breast, and prostate. All can spread to the liver. Lymphomas and sometimes leukemias can also involve the liver.

Treatment options depend upon the type of cancer. Patients with cancers that arise in the liver, namely hepatocellular carcinomas or cholangiocarcinomas, generally have bad outcomes. Very small tumors of these types may be able to be resected surgically or treated by liver transplantation with a chance of cure. Usually, however, the cancer is fairly large at the time of diagnosis. For any scenario, various treatment options exist such as alcohol injection and a technique known as *emoblization,* which causes disruption of the tumor's blood supply. These usually do not cure the patient but may alleviate symptoms and prolong life.

Patients with carcinomas from other organs that have spread to the liver almost always have a bad prognosis. Once a carcinoma has spread to the liver from another organ, it is likely disseminated throughout the body. However, some tumors may respond to chemotherapy and rare ones (e.g., testicular) are curable. Other tumors may respond to direct infusion of chemotherapy into the liver. In general, chemotherapy may prolong life or quality of life but not cure the patient with metastatic liver cancer. One notable exception that can be cured is testicular cancer. Lymphoma or leukemia involving the liver may also respond to chemotherapy and be cured.

The bottom line is that patients with "liver cancer" need an extensive workup to establish the type of cancer and the extent to which it might have already spread (metastasized) throughout the body. Treatment options can then be considered. Unfortunately, the prognosis is not good for *most* types of cancer that involve the liver. Patients with liver cancers should generally be evaluated by an oncologist or medical cancer specialist to determine appropriate treatment options.

Q: I have fatty liver. Who can I see to make the fat go away?

A: Fat most frequently infiltrates the liver of individuals who drink alcohol, those with diabetes mellitus, and obese individuals. Some drugs can also cause fat in the liver. Occasionally, fat can be seen in the liver of otherwise apparently healthy individuals. The diagnosis is usually *suspected* when ALT and/or AST activities are elevated on blood tests and there is no other obvious cause of liver disease. The diagnosis of fatty liver can be made only by liver biopsy. There are two major forms of fatty liver distinguished on liver biopsy. One, called *steatosis,* is only the presence of fat within the liver. The other, more severe form is called *steatohepatitis* and is characterized by fat plus a particular type of inflammation. Steatosis generally has a good prognosis but steatohepatitis can progress to cirrhosis. If the cause of steatohepatitis is not alcohol-related, it is sometimes called *"non-alcoholic steatohepatitis"* or *"NASH."*

If alcohol is the cause of fatty liver, the patient should stop drinking, and fatty liver will thereupon reverse. If a drug is suspected, the drug should be discontinued (by the doctor, *not* the patient). Although there are no large, well-controlled studies, clinical experience and common sense suggest that fatty liver will resolve in obese individuals who lose weight. A healthy, low-fat diet and exercise may also help non-obese individuals with fatty liver. For diabetics who have fatty liver, better control of blood sugar may help it resolve. So, either less or no alcohol, a low-fat diet, exercise, weight loss in overweight individuals, and better control of blood sugar in diabetics may help eliminate the fat in individuals with fatty liver.

Q: I have a liver disease not related to alcohol. Can I drink?

A: This is a tough question. There is no definite right or wrong answer and no scientific data on which to base a decision (except to state the obvious: Excessive drinking *is* dangerous). Some liver specialists strongly believe that patients with any liver disease should *never* drink alcohol. Others, myself included, feel that *reasonable* alcohol intake is most likely not harmful. (However, I feel strongly that patients with alcoholic liver disease, or those with alcohol abuse or dependency disorders, should *never* drink alcohol.)

My teacher, Dr. Fenton Schaffner, a distinguished liver specialist, used to tell his patients with *nonalcoholic* liver diseases
that it was okay to drink as long as they consumed "only the
good stuff." His point was that a small quantity of responsible
drinking is probably not harmful. A couple of glasses of wine
with a nice dinner, a beer at the ballgame, a glass of champagne
at a party, or an occasional cocktail will probably do little harm.
I can't provide an exact number regarding how many drinks
would be considered excessive for individuals with liver disease,
but definitely not more than two drinks per day on a regular
basis. My general recommendation is that mild alcohol intake is
probably safe for most individuals with liver diseases, except, of
course, for persons with alcoholic liver disease or a substance
use disorder. Again, not all liver specialists agree and some will
state that patients with liver disease should never drink.

Q: I have a liver problem and my doctor or HMO refuses to
send me to a specialist. Can you please help me?

A: Most general internists, pediatricians, and family doctors
should be able to diagnose the most common liver diseases. If
you really think that your doctor cannot, it is an unfortunate
situation and I can only recommend going to another doctor. I
don't know what to say if your HMO or insurance provider
does not allow you to see another doctor, except to explore
your legal options by contacting a state medical board, state insurance board, or attorney.

Problems sometimes arise with specialized treatments, the
diagnosis of rare diseases, and liver transplantation. Sometimes,
a small HMO may not have a doctor who knows how to diagnose, treat, and manage patients with rare liver disorders such as
primary biliary cirrhosis, autoimmune hepatitis, or Wilson disease. Sometimes, doctors in HMOs or rural communities really

do not know when to refer patients for liver transplantation (although in today's society, I hope that most do). I do not know exactly how to help, except to recommend that you explore legal options if your HMO or insurance provider prohibits a second opinion by a specialist. The bottom line is that life comes before money, and in some cases a patient's only option may be to pay cash for a onetime second opinion consultation with a liver specialist not covered by insurance. In many cases, you will be relieved to hear that your current doctor is doing things correctly (this will probably be worth the cost of one visit for most patients). If by chance you learn that your current doctor cannot handle the problem, a letter from an outside expert explaining why you need specialized treatment not available in your "network" *may* help to convince your HMO to change its opinion about covering outside care.

Q: What can I do to lower my liver enzymes?

A: The goal for a patient with a liver disease is *not* to treat laboratory values. The goal is to make a diagnosis to determine the cause of the laboratory abnormality. Then specific treatments or interventions aimed at the disease and not the laboratory abnormality can be prescribed. Absolute values of so-called liver enzymes (generally blood ALT, AST, alkaline phosphatase, and GGTP activities) are not the major issue. Identification and treatment of the disease is.

Resources

Many patients want disease-related information that goes far beyond the scope of this book. Some even want to read medical textbooks or stay up-to-date with the latest medical literature. Major breakthroughs in medicine related to liver disease will probably be reported by the major television networks. Newspapers such as the *New York Times* or *Wall Street Journal* frequently report major findings. Medical news concerning new drug treatments that influence pharmaceutical companies is often reported in the business sections of major American newspapers.

For the lay person who really wants to learn about liver diseases in depth, or keep up with the most current literature, following are the names of the major textbooks on liver disease and relevant major medical journals. Given that more and more people are surfing the Web for medical information, I have provided some Internet resources that I feel are reputable. Please note that these lists are not complete but merely represent my personal recommendations.

Medical Textbooks Aimed at Health Professions

Most doctors start with a textbook when looking for information related to liver diseases. Remember, no textbook is absolutely authoritative, and some are better than others in different areas. Textbooks also become outdated. And finally, books are not gospel—including this one—and information written as fact may be wrong!

There are numerous textbooks devoted to internal medicine and pediatrics. There are others focusing specifically on liver diseases. The best way to find a good one is to visit a medical school library and ask for one that is kept "on reserve" at the front desk. These are likely to be the most up-to-date. Because they are very expensive, I do not recommend buying one unless you are a physician or medical student.

Medical and Scientific Journals

Basic discoveries that will ultimately become important in liver diseases may be published in highly technical journals. These papers are usually incomprehensible to nonspecialists and even most practicing physicians. However, some scientific journals will publish papers that may have an immediate impact on clinical liver disease, for example, the cloning of a gene that causes a particular genetic disease or the discovery of a new hepatitis virus. Some of these high-impact general scientific journals are:

American Journal of Human Genetics (genetic diseases)
Cell (general)
Genomics (genetic diseases)
Immunity (immune system/autoimmune)
Journal of Biological Chemistry (biochemistry of liver/diseases)
Journal of Cell Biology (cell biology of liver/diseases)
Journal of Clinical Investigation (general)
Journal of Experimental Medicine (mostly immune system/ autoimmune)
Journal of Immunology (immune diseases/autoimmune)
Journal of Virology (hepatitis viruses)
Nature (general)
Nature Genetics (genetic diseases)
Nature Medicine (general)
Proceedings of the National Academy of Sciences USA (general)
Science (general)

The most significant clinical papers related to liver diseases that will impact on clinical practice will usually be published in the most important general medical journals including:

Annals of Internal Medicine
Lancet
New England Journal of Medicine

There are also several specialized journals that publish papers on both clinical hepatology and science related to liver diseases. Some of the more important of these specialized "liver journals" are:

American Journal of Gastroenterology
Gastroenterology
Gut
Hepato-gastroenterology

Hepatology
Journal of Hepatology
Journal of Viral Hepatitis
Liver

Reputable Internet Resources

Many patients, friends, and family members are turning to the Internet, especially the World Wide Web, for medical information and even advice. When using the Internet, *be careful*. Anyone can put up an impressive-looking Website and make ridiculous or misleading information seem important. Many also try to sell miracle cures or wonder treatments that the medical profession has ignored or tried to suppress (watch out for these!). People can masquerade as doctors and professors and provide medical advice. My strongest recommendation is *never accept medical advice from anyone except a doctor who has taken a complete medical history and examined you.* There are literally thousands of medical Websites. I will provide only a brief list and accompanying description of the few with information on liver diseases that I consider to be not only the best but reputable. Again, I apologize to the creators of Websites I have omitted that are quite good. Some of the liver-related Websites that I recommend are:

Alcohol-Related

Al-Anon and Alateen
http://www.Al-Anon-Alateen.org/

This Website is the work of Al-Anon member volunteers in various countries. It provides information about this organization for family members and friends of individuals with alcohol use disorders.

Alcoholics Anonymous
http://www.alcoholics-anonymous.org
Website of Alcoholics Anonymous (AA). It contains information about AA and how individuals with alcohol use disorders can obtain additional materials.

General Liver Disease Information

American Association for the Study of Liver Diseases
http://hepar-sfgh.ucsf.edu/
Homepage of the predominant American organization for physicians and biomedical scientists with an interest in the liver and its diseases.

American Liver Foundation
http://www.liverfoundation.org/
The American Liver Foundation is a national, voluntary health agency dedicated to preventing, treating, and curing hepatitis and all liver diseases.

Current Papers in Liver Disease
http://cpmcnet.columbia.edu/dept/gi/references.html
Part of my "Diseases of the Liver" site that comprises an annotated list of recent papers that relate to diseases of the liver. It is not an extensive review of all papers published but a few selections considered either to be of outstanding significance or to have a possible impact on clinical care.

Diseases of the Liver
http://cpmcnet.columbia.edu/dept/gi/disliv.html
My own site at Columbia University.

National Institute of Diabetes and Digestive and Kidney Diseases (NIDDK)
http://www.niddk.nih.gov/
NIDDK is the institute of the U.S. National Institutes of Health which is devoted to most issues regarding digestive diseases. This site contains information on digestive diseases, research funding, and NIDDK's own intramural research programs and clinical trials.

Liver Pathology

Dr. Greenson's Gastrointestinal and Liver Pathology
http://www.pds.med.umich.edu/users/greenson/
The homepage of Dr. Joel Greenson at the University of Michigan devoted to gastrointestinal and liver pathology. One of the first Websites devoted to liver diseases, and a lot of fun.

Hepatic Pathology Index (Webpath)
http://www.medlib.med.utah.edu/WebPath/LIVEHTML/LIVERIDX.html
Excellent pictures of gross and microscopic liver pathology. Created by Dr. Edward C. Klatt at the University of Utah.

Liver Transplantation and Childhood Liver Diseases

American Share Foundation
http://www.asf.org/index.html
A large nonprofit organization that provides information on liver transplantation, especially as it relates to children.

Children's Liver Alliance
http://www.livertx.org/
Support groups of children (and their parents) with liver diseases.

United Network for Organ Sharing (UNOS)
http://www.unos.org
UNOS administers the national Organ Procurement and Transplantation Network and the Scientific Registry on Organ Transplantation under contracts with the U.S. Department of Health and Human Services. The site contains information on liver transplantation.

Metabolic Liver Diseases

Online Mendelian Inheritance in Man (OMIM)
http://www3.ncbi.nlm.nih.gov/Omim/
OMIM is a comprehensive database of human genes and genetic disorders authored and edited by Dr. Victor A. McKusick and his colleagues at Johns Hopkins University. Developed for the World Wide Web by the National Center for Biotechnology Information (NCBI), it is arguably the best online resource on inherited liver diseases such as Wilson disease, familial hemochromatosis, and alpha-1-antitrypsin deficiency.

Searching the Medical Literature

National Center for Biotechnology Information Pub Med
http://www.ncbi.nlm.nih.gov/PubMed/
This Website provides the user with access to free searches of the primary literature. Abstracts are available for many articles.

Viral Hepatitis

Hepatitis Branch Homepage Centers for Disease Control and Prevention (CDC)

http://www.cdc.gov/ncidod/diseases/hepatitis/index.htm
The homepage of the Hepatitis Branch of the CDC, the U.S. government organization whose mission is the control of infectious diseases.

HepNet

http://www.hepnet.com/
A comprehensive site with lots of excellent information on viral hepatitis. For possible conflict-of-interest purposes, I should point out that the person who created and maintains this site is an employee of Schering-Plough, a company that sells drugs for the treatment of viral hepatitis.

Management of Hepatitis C (National Institutes of Health Consensus Development Conference Statement)

http://odp.od.nih.gov/consensus/cons/105/105_statement.htm
Complete text of the U.S. National Institutes of Health Consensus Development Conference Statement of March 24–26, 1997, on the management of hepatitis C. An important document. Some of it, however, especially treatment issues, is outdated.

Glossary

This glossary is used to define words found throughout the book that are related to the liver and its diseases. The names of specific liver diseases are not included in the glossary. For information concerning them, see the appropriate chapters in which they are discussed.

Activity – A unit of measurement used by biochemists that is proportional to the amount of an enzyme at a given temperature, concentration, and other conditions. Various blood tests used to assess liver function are measured in units of activity.

Albumin – The most abundant protein in the blood that is synthesized in the liver. Its concentration in the blood may be low when liver function is compromised.

Alcohol use disorders – Conditions precisely defined in the American Psychiatric Association's *Diagnostic and Statistical Manual of Mental Disorders* that describe people with chronic problems related to alcohol consumption. The chronic alcohol use disorders are alcohol abuse and alcohol dependency.

Alcoholic – An ill-defined term applied to a person with either an alcohol abuse or alcohol dependency disorder.

Alkaline phosphatase – An enzyme present in the bile ducts, as well as other organs such as bone, kidney, and placenta. Its activity is frequently measured in the blood and elevations may indicate bile duct or liver disease.

ALT – See Aminotransferases.

Aminotransferases – Enzymes present in hepatocytes (and other tissues). The activities of two aminotransferases, alanine aminotransferase (ALT) and aspartate aminotransferase (AST), are frequently measured in the blood. These enzymes leak out of hepatocytes when they are damaged or die. Their blood activities are often elevated in liver diseases such as hepatitis.

Antibodies – Proteins in the blood that are produced by cells of the immune system and which recognize components of infecting organisms such as viruses or bacteria. In abnormal circumstances, the immune system may make antibodies against the body's own components. These antibodies are called autoantibodies.

Antigen – A protein or other type of chemical compound recognized by an antibody (see also Antibodies).

Antimitochondrial antibodies – A type of autoantibody found in the large majority of patients with primary biliary cirrhosis (see also Autoantibodies).

Antinuclear antibodies – Types of autoantibodies found in patients with various autoimmune liver diseases such as primary biliary cirrhosis, primary sclerosing cholangitis, and autoimmune hepatitis (see also Autoantibodies).

Ascites – Abnormal accumulation of edema fluid in the abdomen (see also Edema).

AST – See Aminotransferases.

Autoantibodies – Antibodies against components of an individual's own body (see also Antibodies).

Autoimmune – A state in which the body's immune system attacks and damages tissues and organs. Primary biliary cirrhosis, primary sclerosing cholangitis, and autoimmune hepatitis are thought to be autoimmune liver diseases.

Autosomal recessive disorders – Genetic diseases in which two abnormal copies of a gene must be inherited for the disease to be manifested. The liver diseases hereditary hemochromatosis, alpha-1-antitrypsin deficiency, and Wilson disease are autosomal recessive disorders.

Bilirubin – A chemical compound produced in the human body primarily due to the breakdown of old red blood cells. It is taken up by the liver, changed to a more soluble form, and then secreted into the bile. The blood bilirubin concentration is often measured in a clinical laboratory and may be elevated in various liver diseases, as well as in some conditions in which red blood cells are destroyed at an abnormal rate. If the blood bilirubin concentration is higher than about 2 mg per deciliter, the person will appear jaundiced.

bDNA – A type of blood test sometimes used to measure the amount of hepatitis C viral RNA in the blood.

Cachexia – A generalized wasting, especially of muscle mass, that is evidenced in advanced cirrhosis as well as other chronic diseases.

CAT scan – Computerized axial tomography; an X-ray test used to obtain cross-sectional images of the body. It may be useful in evaluating the liver and gallbladder, especially when searching for tumors, gallstones, or evidence of bile duct obstruction.

Cholestasis – Stagnation of bile flow in the liver.

Conjugation – The chemical reaction in bilirubin metabolism in which glucuronic acid moieties couple with bilirubin to make it soluble so that it can be secreted into the bile. Conjugation takes place in hepatocytes of the liver and is catalyzed by the enzyme UDP-glucuronosyltransferase. Other substances, such as drugs and toxins, may also be conjugated in the liver to make them more soluble for elimination either in the bile or by the kidneys.

CT scan – See CAT scan.

Edema – Abnormal accumulation of fluids in the tissues of the body.

Encephalopathy – Abnormal mental functioning secondary to organic causes (see Hepatic encephalopathy).

Endoscope – A fiber-optic tube used to visualize the inside of body cavities, including the upper and lower gastrointestinal tract. For patients with liver diseases, endoscopy may be necessary to visualize the esophagus, stomach, or proximal small intestine. These tubes may be modified so that procedures can be performed through them under direct visualization.

Endoscopic retrograde cholangiopancreatography (ERCP) – A procedure in which a small tube in inserted into the bile via an endoscope and dye is injected. An X-ray image can then be obtained of the bile ducts inside and outside the liver as well as the pancreatic duct because X-rays cannot pass through the injected dye. This procedure can also be modified to conduct procedures, such as removing gallstones trapped in a large bile duct.

Endoscopic rubber band ligation – A procedure in which esophageal, or possibly gastric, varices are tied off through a fiber-optic tube (endoscope) under direct visualization.

Endoscopic sclerotherapy – A procedure in which esophageal varices are treated with a caustic chemical to occlude them. This procedure is performed via a fiber-optic tube (endoscope) under direct visualization.

Enlarged liver – See Hepatomegaly.

Enzyme – A protein that catalyzes (speeds up) a chemical reaction.

ERCP – See Endoscopic retrograde cholangiopancreatography.

Esophageal varices – Varicose veins in the esophagus.

Fibrosis – Scar tissue.

First pass metabolism – A term used to describe the chemical reactions that many drugs and toxins undergo in the liver before reaching the systemic circulation (matter absorbed in the gut go first to the liver before they reach the heart).

Gamma-glutamyltranspeptidase – Often abbreviated as GGTP, it is an enzyme present in the bile ducts. Its activity in the blood is frequently measured in the clinical laboratory. Elevations can indicate a wide variety of liver diseases and may be high in some individuals without any significant disease. It may be elevated in patients who consume excess alcohol or are taking certain drugs. It may also indicate bile duct disease.

Gastric varices – Varicose veins in the stomach.

Gastroenterologist – A doctor who specializes in diseases of the digestive system, including the liver. Some gastroenterologists, however, prefer to care primarily for patients with diseases of the esophagus, stomach, intestines, and rectum and do not devote much time to liver diseases.

Genotypes – Slightly different strains of the hepatitis C virus that are classified based upon the sequences of their genetic material.

GGTP – See gamma-glutamyltranspeptidase.

Gynecomastia – Breast enlargement in men that can occur as a result of cirrhosis and poor metabolism of circulating estrogens in the blood.

HBIG – See Immune globulin.

Hepatic encephalopathy – A change in mental state caused by the liver's inability to metabolize ammonia and other nitrogen-containing toxins absorbed from the gut that are toxic to the brain. Clinically, hepatic encephalopathy can range from subtle changes in the ability to concentrate to a deep coma.

Hepatic artery – A blood vessel that delivers oxygen-rich blood to the liver directly from the heart.

Hepatic vein – The major vein through which blood exits the liver.

Hepatitis – A general term meaning inflammation of the liver. There are many causes of hepatitis including alcohol, drugs, toxins, viruses, and metabolic disorders.

Hepatocyte – The liver's primary cell type. Many different biochemical reactions essential for whole body metabolism and health take place in hepatocytes.

Hepatologist – A doctor who specializes in diseases of the liver.

Hepatology – The study of liver diseases.

Hepatomegaly – Enlarged liver. It is not specific for any one liver disease. There are many causes including some diseases of the liver.

Hepatorenal syndrome – A type of kidney failure seen only in patients with liver failure. It is virtually always fatal unless liver transplantation is performed.

Heterozygote – Regarding genetic diseases, this term is used to refer to a person who has inherited one copy of an abnormal gene. In autosomal recessive disorders, a heterozygote will not have the disease but would be a carrier.

Homozygote – Regarding genetic diseases, this term is used to refer to a person who has inherited two copies of an abnormal gene. In autosomal recessive disorders, a homozygote will have the disease.

Hyperbilirubinemia – Elevated bilirubin concentration in the blood.

Hypoalbuminemia – Low albumin concentration in the blood.

Immune globulin – A preparation of antibodies against a particular organism. Hepatitis B immune globulin (HBIG) contains antibodies against the hepatitis B virus and may be given to people with known exposure. In general, immune globulin almost always has antibodies against the hepatitis A virus and may be given to people who are exposed to this virus or traveling to high-risk areas before having time to be vaccinated.

Immunosuppressive drugs – A class of drugs used to suppress the immune system and prevent organ transplant rejection. Some are also used to treat autoimmune hepatitis.

Interferon – Naturally occurring substances that have many functions in the body, including helping to fight off viral infections. Synthetic types of interferon, administered by injection, are used in the treatment of hepatitis B and hepatitis C.

Jaundice – Yellowing of the skin, the whites of the eyes, and the mucous membranes secondary to high bilirubin concentrations in the blood.

Kayser-Fleischer rings – Abnormalities seen in the eye in most patients with Wilson disease.

Lamivudine – An orally administered drug approved for the treatment of chronic hepatitis B. It belongs to the class of drugs known as nucleoside analogues.

Liver enzymes – A term used for various blood tests related to the liver. Generally used to refer to aminotransferases, it can also be used to refer to alkaline phosphatase and gamma-glutamyltranspeptidase.

Liver palms – Reddish palms (called palar erythema by doctors) that may be seen in individuals with various liver diseases.

Liver-spleen scan – A nuclear medicine test that can sometimes detect cirrhosis.

MRI scan – Magnetic resonance imaging; an imaging study of the part of the body that utilizes the phenomenon known as nuclear magnetic resonance. It is sometimes used to visualize the liver and may be useful in searching for certain types of tumors.

Paracentesis – A procedure in which fluid (ascites) is removed from the abdominal cavity by inserting a needle through the abdominal wall. A small amount of fluid may be removed for diagnostic purposes or a large amount for therapeutic reasons.

PCR – See Polymerase chain reaction.

Platelets – The smallest blood cells that play a role in blood clotting.

Polymerase chain reaction – A type of chemical reaction used to amplify small amounts of DNA of a specific sequence. This type of chemical reaction, combined with reverse transcription or copying of RNA to DNA, can be used to detect hepatitis C virus RNA in the blood.

Portal gastropathy – Diffusely dilated veins in the stomach that result from portal hypertension.

Portal hypertension – Usually caused by cirrhosis, it is high blood pressure in the portal vein and connected veins. Portal hypertension can lead to many problems including the development of gastric and esophageal varices and splenomegaly.

Portal vein – The major blood vessel that supplies blood to the liver. Blood in the portal vein contains substances absorbed from the stomach and gut.

Prothrombin time – A blood test used to measure the amounts of certain clotting factors in the blood. It may be prolonged if liver function is abnormal. It may also be prolonged in other disorders.

Pruritus – Severe itching, a symptom of some liver diseases.

Quasispecies – Slightly different variants of the hepatitis C virus that arise by mutations in the viral RNA.

Red blood cells – Cells that circulate in the blood whose function is to carry oxygen.

Ribavirin – An orally administered drug used in combination with interferon alpha-2b in the treatment of chronic hepatitis C.

Shunt – A type of surgical procedure in which a vein of the portal circulation is connected to a blood vein of the systemic circulation to relieve portal hypertension. Besides being performed during surgery, a type of shunt is also done by radiologists (see also Transjugular intrahepatic portosystemic shunt).

Sonogram – See Ultrasound.

Spider angiomata – Small marks on the skin denoting central red areas with "legs" that radiate out from the center, making them look like spiders. If pressure is applied, they blanch and turn red again when pressure is released. Observed in patients with chronic liver diseases and sometimes in pregnant women.

Splenomegaly – An enlarged spleen that can be caused by portal hypertension.

Steatosis – Pathologist's term for fatty liver.

Thrombocytopenia – Low platelet count.

TIPS – See transjugular intrahepatic portosystemic shunt.

Transjugular intrahepatic portosystemic shunt – Abbreviated TIPS, it is a procedure performed by radiologists in which a tube is passed through the liver to connect the portal and hepatic veins and reduce portal hypertension. It is indicated to stop bleeding from gastric and esophageal varices.

Ultrasound – An imaging study using sound waves to obtain an image of internal organs. Often used to image the liver and gallbladder, it is an excellent test to detect liver tumors, gallstones, and bile duct obstruction.

Vena cava – The largest vein in the body that returns blood to the heart. The hepatic vein, through which blood exits the liver, empties directly into the vena cava.

Index

About the Author

Howard J. Worman, M.D., is Associate Professor of Medicine and Anatomy and Cell Biology at the College of Physicians and Surgeons at Columbia University. He is also Director of the Division of Digestive and Liver Diseases in the Department of Medicine at Columbia. He received an A.B. cum laude in biology and chemistry from Cornell University and his M.D. from the University of Chicago. Dr. Worman did residency training in internal medicine at New York Hospital and postdoctoral research in cell biology at Rockefeller University. After a stint as an assistant professor at Mount Sinai School of Medicine, where he obtained clinical training in liver diseases, Dr. Worman moved to Columbia University. An author of numerous medical and scientific papers, Dr. Worman is also the creator of the "Diseases of the Liver" World Wide Website (http://cpmcnet. columbia.edu/dept/gi/disliv.html). His laboratory research focuses on basic cancer cell biology, hepatitis C virus infection, and autoimmune liver diseases. His clinical research focuses primarily on the treatment of chronic hepatitis C.